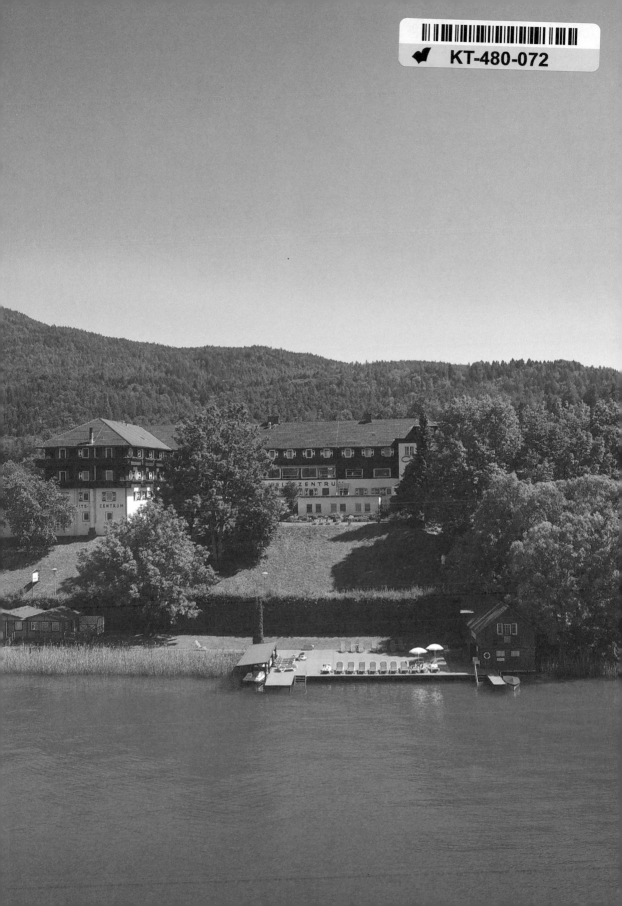

First published in Great Britain in 2014 by

Modern Books, an imprint of Elwin Street Productions Limited

14 Clerkenwell Green

London EC1R 0DP

www.modern-books.com

ISBN 978-1-91113-018-5

10 9 8 7 6

Printed in China

Disclaimer: The advice, recipes and meal plans in this book are intended as a personal guide to healthy living. However, this information is not intended to provide medical advice and it should not replace the guidance of a qualified physician or other healthcare professional. Decisions about your health should be made by you and your health-care provider based on the specific circumstances of your health, risk factors, family history and other considerations. See your healthcare provider before making major dietary changes or embarking on an exercise programme, especially if you have existing health problems, medical conditions or chronic diseases. The author and publishers have made every effort to ensure that the information in this book is safe and accurate, but they cannot accept liability for any resulting injury or loss or damage to either property or person, whether direct or consequential and howsoever arising.

Reprinted by permission: as quoted on page 1

Seven Pillars of Health, Dr Don Colbert, January 2007, Siloam, Charisma House, Florida. All rights reserved.

Front cover: Jason Loucas © Getty

Back cover: Alison Miksch © Getty

THE ALKALINE CURE

DR STEPHAN DOMENIG

Medical Director, The Original F.X. Mayr Health Center

CONTENTS

Introduction
Dr Stephan Domenig, Medical Director,
The Original F.X. Mayr Health Center   8

Section 1: What Is the Alkaline Cure?
What Is the Alkaline Cure?   12
The pH Science Behind the Cure   14
What Causes Excess Acid in the Body?   16
How the Alkaline Cure Can Help You   21
Balance Equals Beauty   25

Section 2: Why You Need the Alkaline Cure
Habits of a Western Lifestyle   28
From the Inside Out   32
When Your System Doesn't Run Smoothly   36
Eat Well, Live Well, Age Well   39

Section 3: Principles of the Alkaline Cure
Guiding Principles of the Alkaline Cure   44
Be Mindful   46
How to Eat   48
What to Eat   50
When to Eat   52
How Much to Eat   53
Stay Hydrated   54
Exercise Regularly   56
Cleanse Your System   57
Enrich Your Surroundings   59
Find Your Rhythm   60

Section 4: Preparing To Go Alkaline

An Alkaline Way of Life   64

Acid Food Groups   67

Alkaline Food Groups   70

Top Alkaline Superfoods   80

The Alkaline Kitchen   84

Section 5: The Fourteen-Day Alkaline Cure

Getting Started   96

Week One Shopping List   100

Days One to Seven   102

Building on Your Cure   116

Week Two Shopping List   118

Days Eight to Fourteen   120

After the Cure   134

Section 6: The Recipes

Teas and Infusions   138

Soups   142

Spreads   148

Breakfast   150

Lunch   153

Dinner   164

Oils, Sauces and Dressings   168

Frequently Asked Questions   170

Recipe Finder   173

Index   174

Acknowledgements   176

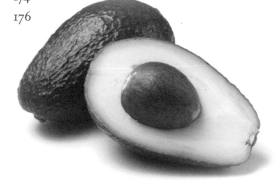

INTRODUCTION

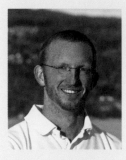

Dr Stephan Domenig
Medical Director
The Original F.X. Mayr
Health Center

I first studied medicine over twenty-one years ago. I was interested in people – why they behave the way they do, how they function and how and why they might be healthy or not. That last question was really the most difficult. Medical school told me everything I wanted to know about diseases and illnesses from a genetic or biochemical standpoint, but there was nothing about what it means to be healthy. Everything was focused on illness. I wanted to know what makes us feel good, but that was just not on the curriculum. The medicine I was taught was a downhill ski run all the way until you died. There was no going back.

Food was not mentioned. Neither was exercise. No one seemed interested in discovering the soul of an illness. I was fascinated by the more holistic approaches – the beauty of the whole body – and I was inspired by ancient health-promoting techniques like Qi Gong and yoga. Medicine, for me, had to be more than just cutting up bodies and tying up bandages.

When I worked in geriatrics, it was all about prolonging life, not the quality of that life. If someone reached one-hundred years old it was celebrated as a big success, never mind that they might not have got out of bed in fifteen years.

Then, over in the metabolic diseases (internal medicine) department there were a few pills and machines that could alleviate patients' suffering in the short term, but those methods were not what I would call medicine. There were very few attempts at understanding or trying anything different.

My first escape from this came with an inspiring course in chiropractic. There, I could use my hands to feel and touch the diseases – realign the spine, improve joint movements. This was fine at the time but I was still not treating the whole body. Then a friend gave me a book written in 1921 called *Fundamentals of the Diagnosis of Digestive Illnesses* by Dr Franz Xaver Mayr.

Mayr explained very elegantly the complete physiology of digestion, its central role for well-being and the connection between tissue tone and function, inner health and posture as one way to evaluate health. It was the first explanation that seemed right in principle – in medicine. I trained to become a Mayr doctor. I have now worked and treated thousands of patients. We combine old knowledge with a modern understanding of the body's biochemistry, its needs for certain nutrients and how what we eat and the way that we eat fundamentally influence our health.

Our approach to well-being centres around one keyword – balance. In the muscles, it's tension and relaxation. For food, it's alkaline and acid in a ratio of 2:1.

The modern Western diet, the ways we choose to eat and our lifestyles tend to encourage an acid overload – high-stress jobs, high-intensity exercise, and last but not least, high-protein diets. Finding our way back to equilibrium is a great chance to improve overall health. That's what the cure is all about.

Our two-week programme is a starting point, an introduction to being your own doctor. It is one that has helped a great many people. And it will help you, too.

Stephan Domenig
Lake Wörthersee, Austria

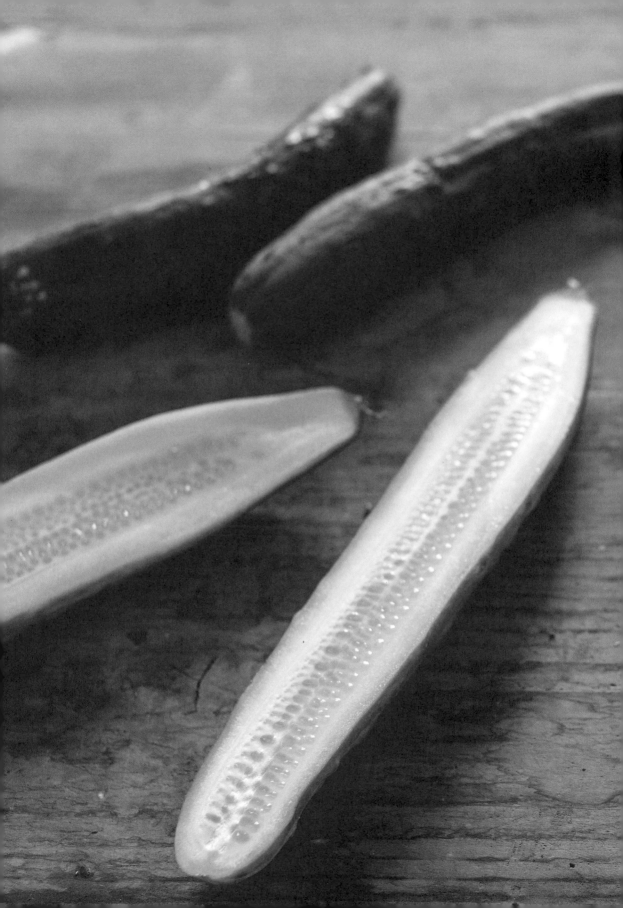

1

What Is the Alkaline Cure?

What Is the Alkaline Cure?
The pH Science Behind the Cure
What Causes Excess Acid in the Body?
How the Alkaline Cure Can Help You
Balance Equals Beauty

WHAT IS THE ALKALINE CURE?

The alkaline cure is a holistic approach to health and well-being. It is a set of simple but powerfully effective diet and lifestyle principles that will bring your digestive system into balance and your body back to its naturally healthy state. These are principles that anyone can follow.

How often do you eat quickly or on the run or late in the evening? And how often do you feel tired, lacking in energy and with a gassy, bloated stomach? These are sure signs your body is suffering from too much acid. The alkaline cure is the solution. It will recharge you and reset your metabolism so that you can experience the energy levels you used to enjoy in the past.

The benefits of the cure are both marked and swift. Regardless of your age and general level of health, if you follow the principles and the plan we give you in this book, you will begin to see results within two weeks. And, if you purchase a pH testing kit and test yourself regularly, you can check those results yourself.

The cure is a powerful anti-ageing programme that will transform you from the inside out. The first benefits tend to be weight loss, increased vitality and improved complexion, skin tone and hair lustre – which is why it is often been called a beauty cure. It will also reward you with stronger bones, better moods, enhanced brain function and a stronger immune system.

The alkaline cure is not a weight-loss programme, although that may be one of its most popular benefits. The aim of the programme is to help you to find your natural, healthy body weight. Your body wants to be healthy; it used to be healthy. You can achieve that by cleaning your system of toxins and identifying the foods and habits that will help you to perform better.

WHERE IT ALL BEGAN

For more than one hundred years, the teachings laid down by the great Dr Franz Xaver Mayr have formed the basis of one of the most effective diet and health regimes in Europe. In that time, Mayr doctors have successfully treated tens of thousands of patients. Mayr, who was born in Austria in 1875, pioneered a radical new approach to wellness.

One of Mayr's pupils, Dr Eric Rauch, opened the first Mayr health clinic in Dellach, on Lake Wörthersee in Austria. This clinic is now known as The Original F.X. Mayr Health Center. It has been much admired, much copied and is a source of help to many people.

The alkaline cure described in this book has evolved from the study and research begun by Dr Mayr. It is based on a clinical understanding of the effects different foods have on the digestive system. According to the Mayr philosophy, good digestion is the most important factor determining human health. It is a holistic and preventative approach, which is to say it is not focused on treating any single disease, but on keeping the whole body healthy.

The alkaline approach has evolved over the years as the study of nutrition has shown us new ways to understand how the body deals with the foods we eat. However, the basic principles of the approach in use today, which we describe in section 3, remain the same as those outlined by Dr Mayr. We believe in the science of nutrition; we know that the food we eat and how we eat it can transform our performance.

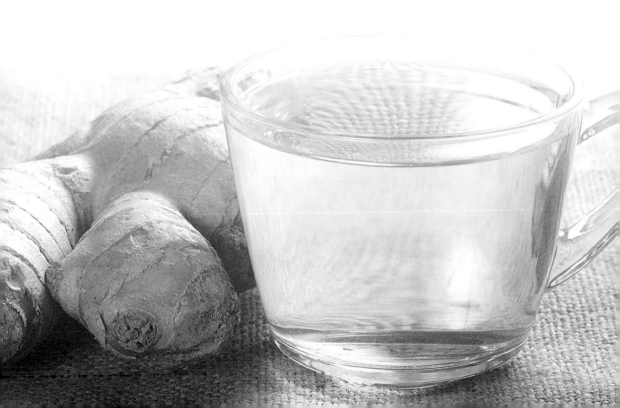

THE PH SCIENCE BEHIND THE CURE

As every farmer knows, you cannot get high yields from a field with acidic (or sour) soil. Just as in nature, so for the human body. At the Original F.X. Mayr & More Health Center we know that in order for the body to be healthy, it needs to have an acid-alkaline balance. How do we know this?

One of the most important methods we use at the health center for evaluating your health is testing your body's pH—in other words, whether your body is acid or alkaline, using the same pH scale that is used by doctors around the world. It is the only single test that gives us an indication of the general health of your body and its systems because the pH of your body's fluids, especially your blood, affects every cell in the body. Keep your body's pH in balance and you will stay healthy.

The beauty of using pH to evaluate health, is that it's as simple as reading numbers. Numbers for pH range from 1 to 14. The higher the pH number the more alkaline you are; 7 is considered neutral and anything below that becomes increasingly acidic. Although 7 is the neutral reading, for optimal health you should be slightly alkaline— ideally around 7.4. This is to counter the increase in acidity that comes with aging and diet.

Be Your Own Doctor

We have provided fourteen test papers and the pH chart at the back of the book to test your body's pH during the cure. We suggest you test yourself on a daily basis at home every morning shortly after you wake up and before eating anything. Don't worry if your initial readings are below 6 and towards the acid end. After two weeks of the cure you will notice a marked improvement. If your reading is already close to 7, that's great. You should still test yourself every day to track changes. Don't be tempted to test yourself more often than daily.

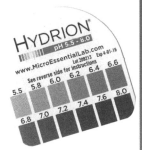

USING THE STRIPS

You can measure your body's pH by using the strips to test your saliva or your urine. It will take longer for the alkalising effect of the cure to reach your urine, so you can generally expect a higher alkaline reading from your saliva. However, testing your urine will give you a more accurate reading as it is a better indicator of how well your kidneys are eliminating acid. Always follow the manufacturer's instructions, and do not put the paper in direct contact with your body.

Saliva

The pH of your saliva is affected by what you have eaten or drunk recently. It is best to wait about two hours after a meal before you test, and then activate and swallow saliva several times to 'rinse' the mouth.

Spit some saliva onto a spoon and dip the litmus paper in the liquid, then compare the resulting colour with the pH colour chart in the packet.

Urine

The pH of your urine is affected by how much water you have consumed and the amount of acid-forming foods you have eaten. For this reason, it is best to test urine first thing in the morning.

Pass a small amount of urine into a cup and dip the litmus paper briefly into the liquid. Compare the result with the pH colour chart in the packet.

(If you would like more test strips you can order these online from Micro Essential Inc., www.microessentiallab.com.)

WHAT CAUSES EXCESS ACID IN THE BODY?

To enable the body to absorb and utilise individual nutrients, the digestive system needs to break down foods appropriately. Unhealthy eating habits, such as eating more food than the digestive system can handle at any one time, cause impaired digestion, which also has a damaging impact on the acid-alkaline balance of the body.

If your pH reading is lower than 7, then it means your body has excess acid. Excess acid in the body is called acidosis. Acidosis occurs when your kidneys and lungs can't keep your body's pH in check (see section 2). Acidosis is much more dangerous than excessive alkalinity (called alkalosis), which is why this cure focuses on how to prevent and reduce excess acidity.

Both the foods you eat and how you eat them may give rise to excess acidity. The modern Western diet means many, or perhaps most of us, eat too much of the wrong kinds of foods (and drink the wrong drinks). Such a diet just clogs up our system and weighs us down.

Lifestyle habits are also a factor, including issues such as stress, lack of sleep, pollution and over-exercising (which causes lactic acid to form). The other major contributor to increasing acidity is age.

PREMATURE AGEING AND ACIDITY

Sagging skin, stiff joints, muscle aches, chronic disease, cognitive deterioration, osteoporosis – we have come to accept these things as a part of growing old, but actually many of these problems are signs that our body is becoming too acidic.

Our modern lifestyles and diets cause us to age faster because we're forcing our bodies to deal with excess acid. In an acidic environment, body cells perform less efficiently and are unable to get rid of toxins. In addition, many health problems are caused by acidic environments. This long list includes irritable bowel syndrome, cardiovascular disease, chronic fatigue, candidiasis, gluten and other food allergies, diabetes and obesity.

Since the body's pH balance is affected by what we eat and how we live, we need to make diet and lifestyle changes in order to reduce

SIGNS THAT YOUR BODY IS TOO ACIDIC

To a trained Mayr doctor, the symptoms of an acidic diet are easy enough to read. These everyday complaints are likely to be symptoms of an acidic diet. Do any of these sound familiar?

Constipation and bloating: Both are caused by eating too fast, too much and/or overly acidic meals.

Lack of energy and focus: Acid depletes blood oxygen availability and you feel sluggish as your brain and systems are deprived of this vital element.

Weight problems: Being overweight suggests that your diet is incompatible with your body's ability to deal with the food it's given.

Poor complexion and dry, dull, lifeless skin: Excess acid is eliminated through the skin, causing skin damage and inflammation.

Gum disease, tooth decay and bad breath: These can be directly related to a high-acid diet, which allows bacteria to develop much more quickly than would occur with an alkaline diet.

Frequent colds and flu: When the body is not being fed the right foods and the flora of the stomach changes, a weak immune system is likely to result.

Muscle and joint pains: Inflammation can be a sign that the alkaline minerals in your bones and muscles are being extracted to neutralise acidity. Particular acids, like arachidonic acid, which is found in red meat, also trigger inflammation.

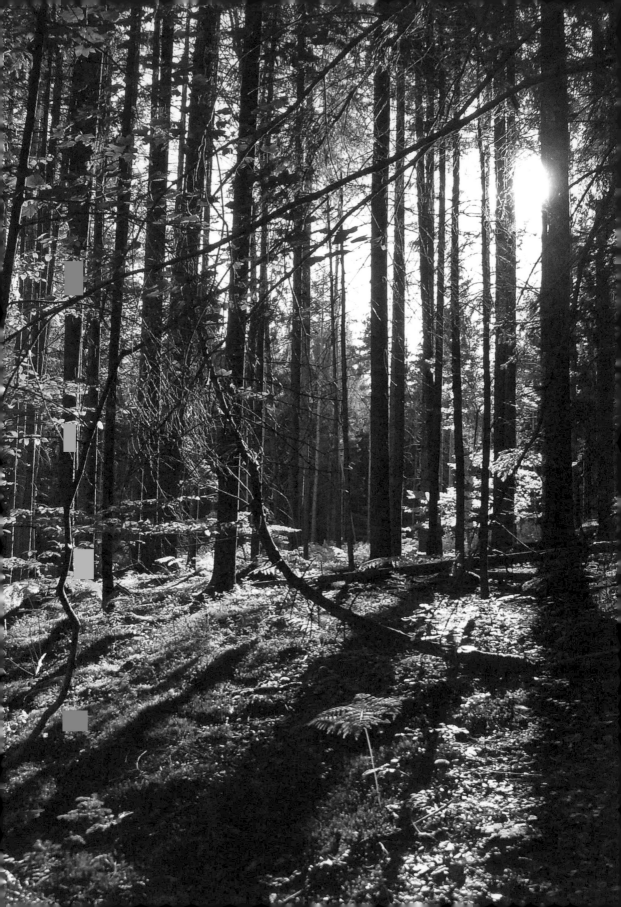

acidity and stay healthy. The single most effective change you can achieve – and the aim of the alkaline cure – is to rebalance your diet by increasing your intake of alkaline foods so that two-thirds of everything you eat is alkaline and only one-third is acid. The aim is to consume foods that taste good, that complement each other and that are easy for your body to digest, thereby maximising your performance. In other words, foods that give you good health.

The 2:1 Alkaline to Acid Rule

In order to increase your alkalinity we do
not suggest only eating alkaline foods. The
best acid-alkaline balance of foods to aim for is two
parts alkaline to a maximum of one part acid. Ideally,
this 2:1 ratio should be on your plate at every meal.
Realistically, this ratio is what you should bear in
mind over the course of your daily and weekly diet.
Be mindful, not fanatical.

Acid in Your Diet

All the foods we eat can be classified as either acid-forming or alkaline-forming, meaning the foods release an acid or alkaline residue during the process of digestion. Note that foods that have an acidic taste (such as lemon, vinegar, rhubarb, etc.) are not necessarily acid-forming. So lemon, while acidic to taste, once digested actually has an alkalising effect on the body. In this book, when we describe foods as 'acid' or 'alkaline', we mean acid-forming or alkaline-forming.

The majority of acid-forming foods are basic staples (see page 67). The more of these foods we eat, the greater the production of acids. The situation can become harmful if the consumption reaches such a level that the metabolism is completely overburdened. There are many different kinds of acid-forming foods that have an effect that varies from strong to weak. The strongest acids are found in animal proteins as well as alcohol, caffeine, processed foods and sugar. The weakest acids are found in vegetable proteins, as present in beans.

Alkaline-forming foods contain very little to no acid and do not produce any acids either. Alkaline foods include most vegetables, many fruits, cold-pressed oils, many grains and all herbs. However, the way we process/digest our food also has an impact on the body. If we eat something alkaline but rush and don't chew properly, it ends up badly digested and ferments, causing acidity.

You can find tables that list acid and alkaline foods in section 4.

The Problem of Protein

Protein is a macro-nutrient composed of amino acids that are necessary for the proper growth and function of the human body. Unfortunately, protein is also one of the most acidic foods, especially animal proteins such as meat and fish (and certain types of cheese). The Food and Agricultural Organization of the United Nations estimates that the amount of protein required by humans is about 20 kilograms for men and 16.5 kilograms for women per year. Britons eat on average about 79.3 kilograms of meat per year while Australians eat over 100 kilograms per year. Most of us (except for serious athletes) eat far too much protein, which results in our bodies becoming protein- and, therefore, acid-saturated. High-protein diets bring with them too much acidity for your stomach to cope with. They may help you lose weight in the short term but will destroy the body's healthy acid/alkaline balance.

A Note on Calories

Over many years different foods have been blamed, correctly or not, for making us fat. The whole conversation about diet has become overloaded with too much emphasis on calories. In this book, we look at diet from a different perspective and use the acid/alkaline monitor, so calories are of less concern. Calories become an issue only because we are sedentary and eat too much. Instead of counting calories, you are better off counting how many times you chew a mouthful of food and ensuring that you get regular exercise.

HOW THE ALKALINE CURE CAN HELP YOU

One of the remarkable things about the alkaline cure is that while acidosis and its effects – the hardening of arteries, the clogging of the digestive system and other bodily malfunctions – may have been building up in your body over the course of many years, the process is swift to reverse. After you have learned the principles of the cure and followed the fourteen-day plan here, you will start to notice a difference. And friends and family will notice, too. But remember, the alkaline cure is not a crash diet but a life plan designed to provide optimal health.

The many benefits of the alkaline cure are extraordinary:

Slows Down the Signs of Ageing

This is the primary and most rewarding benefit of the cure, and one many of the other benefits below also contribute to. We don't promise to stop you ageing, but we do promise to keep you feeling and looking young and staying healthy. One reason that the Mayr alkaline approach has often been labelled as a beauty treatment is that restoring alkalinity to the diet immediately eases many skin, hair and nail problems. Skin regains its youthful radiance and elasticity, hair regains its sheen and nails stop being so brittle. There is little doubt that the alkaline cure can help you to look younger.

Renews Energy and Vitality

You will almost certainly experience renewed vitality as your metabolism improves. Digesting processed, protein-heavy, acid-forming foods requires energy, but without giving back the energy and nutrients it used to process the food. The result is lethargy.

Redressing the acid/alkaline balance corresponds with increased energy as cells have an increased capacity to pass oxygen around the body and so restore vitality. An alkaline diet stabilises energy levels throughout the day, avoiding the highs and lows of sugar rushes from acidic sources such as coffee or refined sugar. By regulating your eating times and changing your diet, you will also feel more energised because you will be sleeping better and deeper.

Encourages Weight Loss

You will lose weight – or, more importantly, achieve your natural body weight or body mass index (BMI). Strictly speaking, the alkaline cure is not a slimming diet. It often helps weight loss because many of us are overweight, but the aim is a healthier you, a better functioning you, a more capable you. Your clearer digestive system and efficient metabolism will lead to weight loss as you eliminate the toxic load you have been carrying. Your renewed energy levels will also motivate you to exercise more so you will become fitter.

Reduces Bloating and Constipation

You will be able to move your bowels regularly and in comfort because you are working with your body, not against it. One very positive sign of good health is passing clear urine and soft faeces. Constipation is bad for you as it stresses your system. An alkaline diet is better than any laxative. If you eat well, you will have a bowel movement every morning. If you drink enough, your stools will be softer. If you chew properly, then the stomach's workload is eased.

Improves Mood and Brain Function

Your mood will improve and you will start to feel more positive and less stressed. In 1987, Rudolph Wiley (PhD), conducted a study in which he postulated that acid imbalance is often a major, and sometimes sole cause of disorders routinely classified as psychological, stress-related, psychosomatic or psychogenic. His study found that an alkaline diet reduced and eliminated the symptom severity in more than 85 per cent of participants.

A broader choice of properly digested food should reduce peaks and troughs in the availability of amino acids and vitamins. Without vitamins such as B6 (from fresh herbs, nuts, legumes, fish), you are likely to experience mood swings and sleeping troubles. The cure also encourages a favourable work-life balance, taking gentle exercise, and the avoidance of alcohol, caffeine and processed food.

In addition to alleviating physical and mental stress, the alkaline cure can help support brain function because it encourages you to eat a diverse range of vitamin- and mineral-rich foods.

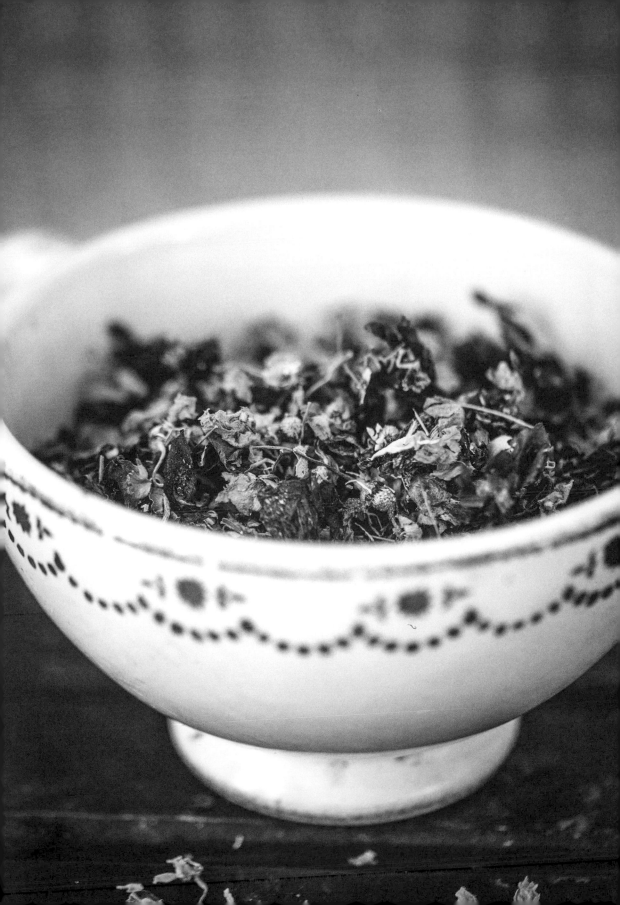

Defends Against Allergy and Disease

Many of our modern-day food allergies are actually the result of inflammation in the stomach. This is seen increasingly in our health clinic when patients react badly to the gluten in wheat and the histamine in aged and fermented foods, milk proteins and, most dramatically, peanuts. The treatment is to identify and avoid the aggravating foods and cleanse the system, giving it a rest from digesting large amounts of food and supplementing the diet with alkalising treatments.

Going beyond allergies, there is compelling scientific research linking diet and the prevalence of chronic conditions such as cancer, heart disease and diabetes. Some theories suggest that these diseases thrive in an acidic environment and are suppressed by an alkaline environment. Additionally, alkaline foods such as vegetables and ripe fruits provide antioxidants, which are a first line of defence against these serious diseases. In essence, the healthier your stomach, the healthier your immune system.

Strengthens Bones

With the alkaline cure, you may find that muscular and skeletal pains start to ease. An alkaline diet can also help prevent, and even treat, osteoporosis as we reduce acidity and support bone formation with alkalising minerals. Healthy bones require an alkaline environment, vitamin D, calcium and weight-bearing exercise.

Increases Fertility

When your body is alkaline and not swamped by acid, the hormonal system slots back into its normal functionality which, in many cases, leads to much greater fertility in men and women. An alkaline environment guarantees better cell function. Many patients at the clinic who thought they could not have children go on to conceive shortly after completing the cure.

BALANCE EQUALS BEAUTY

The alkaline cure is based on a simple premise: regulation of the acid-alkaline balance is an integral part of overall health. The body needs a balance of alkaline and acid foods, in a ratio of two-thirds alkaline and one-third acid, so that overall it is slightly alkaline. Combining acidic and alkaline foods at every meal is the ideal, but may not be practical. If you have eaten a lot of acidic food on an evening out, have an alkaline day the next day to compensate. The key to long-term health is about making small adjustments and developing healthy habits. It really is simple. It really is effective.

Philosophy of Nutrition

The alkaline cure is not a fad diet. There is no calorie counting or gimmicks. It is not about going hungry or going vegetarian, although we do recommend that you eat more vegetables. It isn't strictly a diet at all because it is not about weight loss at the expense of your overall health. The programme is about exchanging bad habits for good ones. It is a philosophy of nutrition that will ensure good health and the maintenance of optimum weight, which is why we describe it as a cure, not a diet.

The alkaline cure is a medically proven approach, based on scientific knowledge from The Original F. X. Mayr Health Center, and has evolved successfully over many decades. It contains everything you need to achieve and maintain balance and vitality in your life, and it will restore your body to its naturally healthy state. For which it will thank you.

It is your body. Be nice to it. Its fate is in your hands.

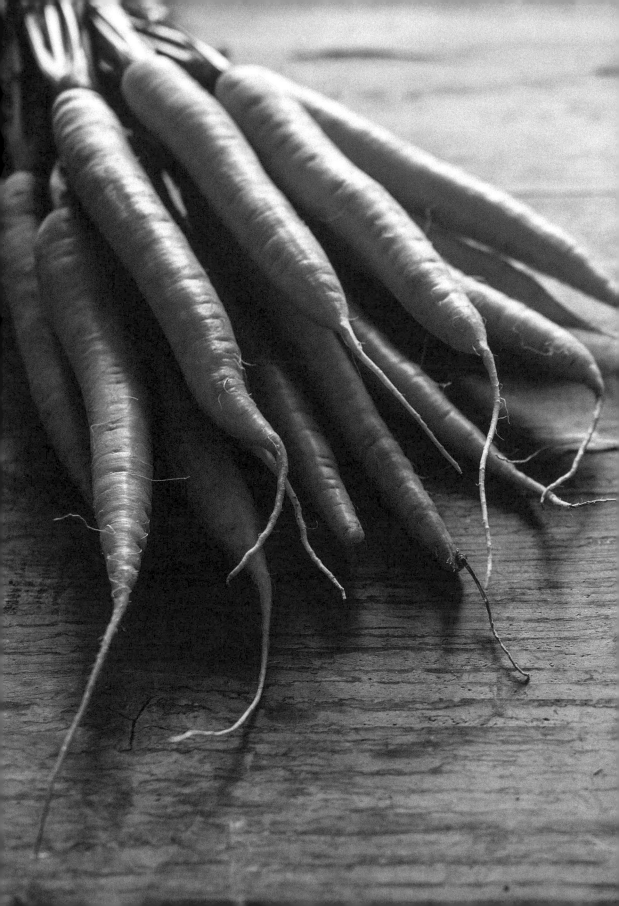

2
Why You Need the Alkaline Cure

Habits of a Western Lifestyle

From the Inside Out

When Your System Doesn't Run Smoothly

Eat Well, Live Well, Age Well

HABITS OF A WESTERN LIFESTYLE

The western world is getting fatter. Take a stroll down any urban high street and the signs and symptoms are there. Over 60 per cent of us are overweight, and over 20 per cent of that number is considered obese. Diabetes rates are at an all-time high – an estimated 4.6 per cent of Britons and Australians have diabetes, the majority with Type 2.

And despite advances in modern medicine, we are still plagued by chronic disease. Most worryingly, our children are getting fatter and they now face a future of health problems. According to a report published by the British government in 2011, 23 per cent of children aged 4–5 and 33 per cent of children aged 10-11 are considered overweight or obese.

In a sense we have forgotten how to eat: we eat too much, we eat the wrong foods and we eat at the wrong times. Overall, we consume too much meat, fish and sugar. We buy too many refined and processed foods that simply fill us up without delivering any real value to help our bodies function. Too much of what we eat has no nutritional value at all – it has been stripped of nutrition through processing before it even gets to us.

Stressing the Diet
The stresses of modern life have encouraged us to see foods as something they are not and to overlook their essential medicinal qualities. Technology has altered the basic things we used to take for granted and depend on, such as bread. We no longer shop at bakers, butchers and fishmongers in local shops where people know what they are selling. Rather, we shop in supermarkets where no one is too sure what they are selling us.

Refined foods such as white bread are now so denatured that they do not deliver any nutritional value and yet still fatten us. Such foods provide only empty calories, taking up space in the stomach that could be occupied by other more useful foods.

Invisible Changes

Overly acidic meals change the shape of the body, which may stop us from exercising properly. We become fatter. But that is just a symptom with its own impact on our health: weighing down our ability to perform physically, overstressing our frames and creating problems for our skeletons. What starts with aches and pains can lead to hip and knee replacements. We become immobilised.

A less visible change is what occurs inside our bodies. Before we get fat, our bones demineralise, our skin sags from lack of nutrients and the toxins we struggle to deal with put strain on our systems. We cope, but we are losing our vitality, our energy, our health.

Toxin Overload

Too much acidity makes us age quicker. Worse, excess acidity creates an environment in the body in which allergies and diseases can flourish. Our digestive tract naturally tries to balance out the mixture of things we consume. The problem is that too much of what we eat is acid-forming and too little is alkaline-forming.

Recovering an Alkaline Balance

How we eat is as important as what we eat. In a busy, modern world the danger is that we often grab food on the go or squeeze meal times into short gaps, and this serves to overload the digestive system. When we eat too quickly we do not give our bodies the chance to digest food fully and absorb the nutrients.

The way our diets have evolved in recent decades – and many of these changes are quite recent – has altered us. What we eat clogs up our systems and weighs us down. These foods stop us from performing at our best, and over time they even change our body shape. We have become accustomed to thinking of everyday foods as healthy when much of what we eat has little nutritional value and just passes through us without delivering any of the minerals or vitamins we need.

Taking Active Steps Towards Health

The answer is not a simple pill, nor to eat more of one particular food. Diets that focus on one element – such as the cabbage soup diet – miss the point. The essential goal should be to redress the overall imbalance. By focusing on how the body performs and eating the right foods, we can regain our strength.

In other words, by cutting down on the acid-forming foods – which in the modern Western diet are largely proteins, refined fats and sugars – and replacing them with more alkalising foods, you can take active steps towards changing your health.

By changing what and how you eat, you may avoid illness in the first place. It is not simply the foods themselves that are at issue but also the body's ability to process them. It is often said that we should be eating a 'balanced diet' without a clear explanation of what that really means in practice.

If you follow the simple ratio of 2:1 alkaline foods to acid, you will achieve that balanced diet. You can revitalise your life by eating a healthier, less acidic, low-protein diet and establishing a positive balance between exercise and rest.

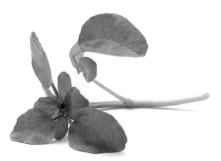

WELCOME TO THE WESTERN DIET

What seems normal and healthy is in fact a menu of
almost continual acidity.

BREAKFAST
Coffee or black tea for breakfast, even without sugar, are acidic.
A croissant for breakfast is also acidic.

SNACK
Biscuits for elevenses are acidic. Cola is acidic. Fruit juice is acidic.
Chocolate bars are acidic.

LUNCH
All the most popular restaurant foods – burgers, pizzas,
fried chicken – are all acidic. A salad might be okay but the dressing
is highly acidic. Even a 'healthy' sandwich and a fizzy drink are acidic, as is
a packet of crisps.

SNACK
In the office, you could top up with still mineral water, a banana and
almonds, but the vending machine does not sell them.

DRINK WITH FRIENDS
By the evening you may feel in need of an alcoholic drink. But a glass of
wine is no real solution. It may make you feel better but it is also acidic.

DINNER
Even a seemingly healthy meal of grilled chicken and salad can be turned
to acid by your high stress levels at the end of the day. Plus you've loaded
up your digestive system with a load of calories just when it thought it
was time to wind down. This will sit with you through the night. And if
you thought pasta or rice was a good idea, you've just put your stomach on
overtime for no gain.

A nice cup of cocoa and a biscuit before you go to bed? More acid.

FROM THE INSIDE OUT

Your nutrition affects everything about you – how fast you age, the condition of your skin, your organs, your energy levels and productivity, your mood and emotions, your weight and, on a grander scale, whether chronic disease will thrive in your body. It has a powerful impact on your quality of life.

At The Original F. X. Mayr Health Center, we believe the digestive system is at the centre of health and well-being. Its role is to process the food we give it – good or bad. The better it functions, the better we function, and the better we look and feel. Nutritionists sometimes talk about a stomach having its own brain. Eating is the last conscious action we take with regard to food. After that our body takes over and decides for itself what it is going to do.

A DAY IN THE LIFE OF YOUR DIGESTIVE SYSTEM

Digestion is the process of breaking down food so that nutrients can be absorbed and used by cells, tissues and organs. A healthy digestive system sets up a rhythm for the day. Each twenty-four hour cycle should, ideally, start with a good breakfast and end the next morning in the toilet. We are all different so the cycle can vary according to what we have eaten and our personal metabolisms.

The Importance of Enzymes

Enzymes are protein-based molecules that start, control and terminate every biochemical process in the body, such as digesting proteins and fats, breaking down and eliminating toxins, neutralising acids, converting food into energy for cells and extracting amino acids from food to build our DNA. There are three categories of enzyme: metabolic (these control each organ and system in our bodies), digestive and food enzymes. Each organ has different enzymes that require specific pH environments to function optimally.

The Role of Saliva

The process of digestion starts in the mouth, where chewing and saliva start to break down starches and protein. Chewing is important for different reasons. First, it allows us to taste and enjoy our food. Secondly, the act of chewing generates more saliva, which is key for digestion. Thirdly, it alerts the rest of the body that food is coming. And masticating and grinding up food, especially proteins such as meat, makes it easier for the rest of the digestive system to perform its role in digestion. If we swallow our food down, or gulp it, or even wash it down with a glass of water, then we are asking the stomach to do all the work, something it is not designed to do.

Saliva helps to maintain a neutral pH in our mouths and provides a reservoir of calcium and phosphate ions to remineralise the teeth and prevent tooth decay. Saliva also contains enzymes that are an essential first step in the digestion of fats and starches, preparing them for processing in other parts of the digestive system. Longer chewing means longer exposure to these enzymes. In addition, saliva is the first contact that any bacteria in the food has with your immune system; if food bypasses the mouth, then it misses the body's first line of defence.

The Role of the Stomach

The stomach is a big acid cauldron that breaks down food as a necessary part of digestion. In order to digest food and kill the kinds of bacteria and viruses that may come with it, the inside of the stomach is acidic with a pH balance of around 1.5. The stomach uses acid and enzymes to break that food into components that are more easily digested in the next stage of the process – which happens in the small intestine.

Roughly speaking, most of us retain food in the stomach for anything from thirty minutes to four hours. However, different foods pass through the stomach at different speeds. Melon, for example, being nearly all water, tends to travel on quickly, while a hunk of beef protein is likely to be kept behind for longer for extra processing. The stomach also produces sodium bicarbonate, which it sends out around the body. Sodium bicarbonate, as well as other bicarbonates, are called 'alkaline buffers' and they help to neutralise excess acid in the body.

The Role of the Small and Large Intestines

An important change occurs in the digestive system between the stomach and the small intestine. The stomach is highly acidic, which it needs to be in order to break up food. When partly digested food passes into the small intestine, your pancreas releases digestive juices that are highly alkaline and that neutralise the acids from the stomach. The pancreatic juices are also rich in enzymes that further break down fats, proteins and carbohydrates.

The main roles of the small intestine are to chemically digest food and absorb nutrients. By the time the food leaves the small intestine, almost every nutrient from it has entered the bloodstream from which the kidneys filter the blood and sieve out any excess water, toxins and acid waste. In order to keep the food residues moving, it is important to drink plenty of fluids; generally speaking, the colour of your urine will be darker if you are not drinking enough fluids and paler if you are drinking a lot. The food residues that remain are passed to the large intestine for further processing.

In the large intestine, the last of the nutritional value is extracted. The major functions of the large intestine are to absorb water from the remaining indigestible food matter, absorb electrolytes, metabolise vitamins and amino acids, and store and excrete waste from the body. This process can take upwards of twelve hours. Once, or sometimes twice, a day it will send the remaining indigestible matter down to the rectum for excretion.

Simplicity and Routine

Just as eating at regular times is good practice, so too is moving your bowels regularly. First thing in the morning is the most obvious time, although for some people it can take a few hours for their bowels to get going after they wake up.

What our stomach wants is a regular life. Simple foods at the right time that don't make it work too hard. In treatments at The Original F. X. Mayr Health Center, we deliberately try to focus on a small range of foods that allow the stomach to reboot itself.

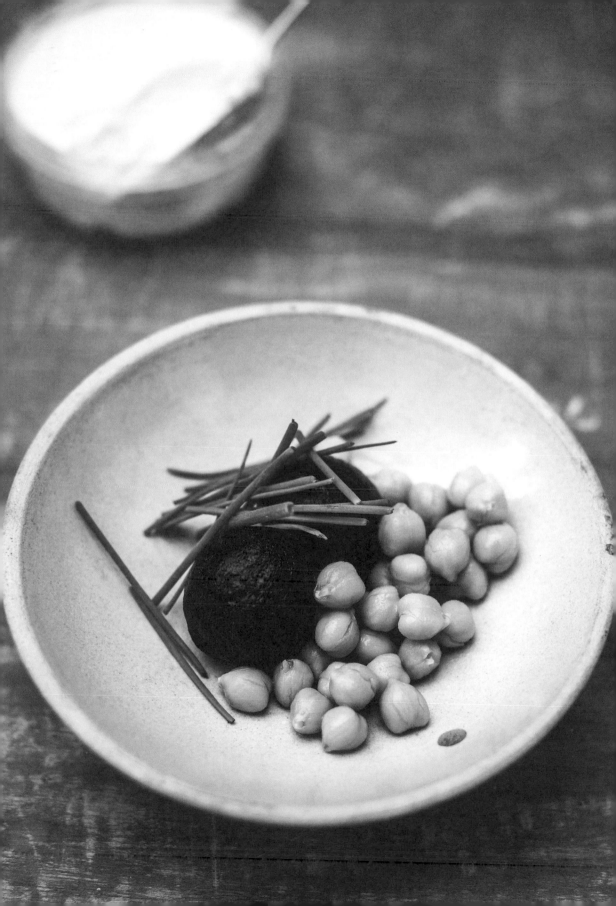

WHEN YOUR SYSTEM DOESN'T RUN SMOOTHLY

Your body is designed to run like an efficient machine, but bad eating habits can wreak havoc on your digestive system. If you eat too fast or too much or too late – or all three – you can overload your digestive system and hamper your stomach's ability to digest.

FERMENTATION

A stomach can only hold and process so much food at a time. If there is more food than it can deal with, the excess food remains in the stomach and putrefy and ferment, eventually moving on with only minor processing. This is made even worse if another batch of food comes along before the stomach is naturally ready, especially if the food being digested is acidic or is taken in late in the evening. As the resulting acids pass down the system they hamper the work of the enzymes that would otherwise translate the mixture into energy and nourishment. In other words, fermentation causes reduced digestive ability, which greatly impacts our overall health and well-being.

Common physical manifestations of putrefaction and fermentation are gas, burping and bad breath. When people complain of 'heartburn', what they should be saying is 'stomach burn' because that is what it is.

Elimination of Acids

Acids produced by metabolic processes in the body are eliminated mainly by the lungs and the kidneys. The carbon dioxide we exhale as we breathe is the quickest way to excrete acid; the alkaline buffers in the kidneys eliminate stomach acids via our urine. Our acid/alkaline balance depends to a large extent on whether these two organs are fulfilling their function of filtering and eliminating properly. Intracellular acidosis, a condition in which your body fluids contain too much acid, occurs when your kidneys and lungs cannot keep the body's pH in balance because the enzymes struggle to digest the food and the alkaline buffers are unable to excrete the acids.

Strong Acids vs Weak Acids

If the digestive system is overloaded with excess acid, not only does this affect the body's cells and enzymes, but also the body has to eliminate the excess in ways that can harm your health. Weak acids (from plant origins) are relatively easy to eliminate from the body by the usual methods. Stronger acids require more work by the kidneys, which have a limited capacity each day to do this, especially as you grow older. Two damaging ways in which the body deals with excess acid involve your skin and bones. Your body can eliminate excess acid through the skin and by sweating, which causes wrinkles, dryness and inflammation. Your body can also leach valuable minerals from your bones in order to neutralise the acids. By depleting the calcium and mineral reserves in your bones, the acids put you at greater risk of developing osteoporosis. This can, however, be prevented by calcium supplements, vitamin D and, most importantly, restoring your acid/alkaline balance through diet.

Acids clearly have a significant impact on the functioning of your whole body, but by redressing the acid/alkaline balance, you will reap the benefits of better-functioning organs, more beautiful and radiant skin, and stronger bones.

Raw Vegetables

Raw vegetables and raw fruits are important alkaline foods, but they are especially prone to fermentation. If you eat most of your fruit and vegetables in raw form, you won't get the alkaline benefit, but instead will become more acidic. Avoid this by staying away from raw food in the evening and not eating more raw foods than the digestive system can properly digest.

THE EFFECTS OF STRESS

The stomach reacts very badly to stress of any kind – emotional or physical. It does not like it. It seizes up and stops functioning as efficiently. If you eat while stressed, the stress signals tell your stomach you're doing something else. You are not eating. Your stomach reacts by halting the digestive process and waiting for things to get better.

Therefore eating when stressed is, nutritionally speaking, a bad idea. The stomach will either hang on to anything it has got or pass it on without doing its normal job. For the same reason, eating on the run is also not a good idea. In both instances, only a small proportion of the nutrients will be extracted.

Modern everyday pick-me-ups such as cola, coffee and alcohol may seem like they help with stress, but they don't. Sugar is the worst culprit, offering a short fix but then disappearing – leaving behind the calories, draining the body's minerals and making us crave for more.

AN AGEING DIGESTIVE SYSTEM

As the body ages, it tends to have more digestive problems because natural supplies of enzymes decrease. Vital digestive processes start to slow and illness results because acid toxins can't be eliminated efficiently, food isn't digested and absorbed properly and energy isn't delivered to the cells.

You may be able to cope with fizzy drinks and chips in your twenties, but over the years the effects become all too visible. You need a diet rich in alkaline foods that can replenish your enzyme stores and help your body combat the symptoms of ageing.

This is just part of the evidence that helped Dr Mayr, and his followers understand that to be healthy and to have a well-functioning metabolism we need to have an efficient digestive system. And that includes eating the right balance of foods. Put simply, we know that if you eat well, you will live well and age well.

EAT WELL, LIVE WELL, AGE WELL

Modern medicine has achieved wonderful breakthroughs, but its achievements should not obscure or divert us away from a simple truth – if we pay attention to, and carefully choose, the foods we eat every day, then we can often avoid going to the doctor in the first place.

Eat Well

Dr Mayr's philosophy was to treat all his patients in the same way. He argued that if the stomach and the digestive system function properly, many diseases would not arise – a healthy body doesn't allow them to flourish.

The power of food to heal the human body is proven in front of our eyes every day at the clinic. We see patients lose weight. We have also seen patients – both men and women – who believed they were infertile but were able to have children after following the dietary advice here. In many cases, stomach pain eases and skin clears – immediate signs pointing to a healthier future. Also central to the Mayr approach is *how* we eat – chewing well and taking your time when eating are crucial to good health.

The past decades have seen an unprecedented increase in fast food consumption and the industrialisation of what we eat. More and more of our food is being processed and loaded with preservatives, flavour enhancers, added sugar and salt. These have a demonstrable ill-effect on our health and well-being. We need to return to eating natural, organic foods that are in season.

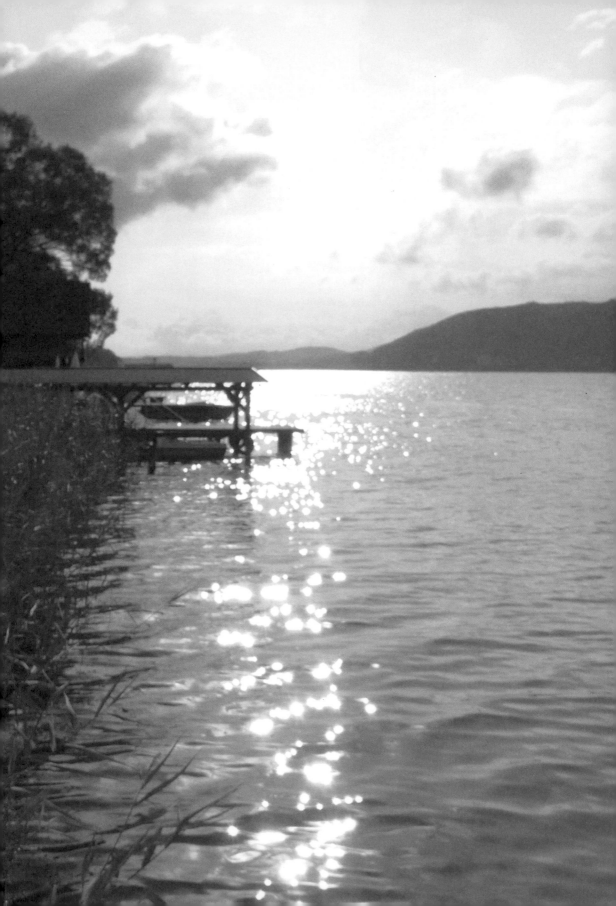

Live Well

However, diet alone is not the answer to good health. Another fundamental part of our approach is a better lifestyle. Gentle cardio and breathing exercises improve blood circulation, strengthen the body and, in turn, support the internal systems and ease stress. Activities that bring you joy – such as dancing, hiking or swimming – or peace – such as yoga or meditation – are also good for us.

Our immediate surroundings are important to our health: open windows bring fresh air; plants and flowers supply oxygen; music soothes and brings happiness.

Age Well

We all grow old but acidic diets and poor lifestyle cause us to age faster than we naturally should. We have come to accept chronic ailments and diseases as a normal part of living. But many symptoms of old age can be postponed by a healthier diet. Most diseases and ailments develop over years. A cup of coffee this morning is not going to kill you. A hamburger is not going to kill you. The long-term effects of these acidic foods – for instance, the leaching of minerals from bones – occur slowly but build up over years.

The advice in this book will put your body back in harmony by eradicating these negative influences and encouraging a change in your eating and lifestyle. Life is always about balance, rhythm and cycles, and the only person who can tell you to take action is you.

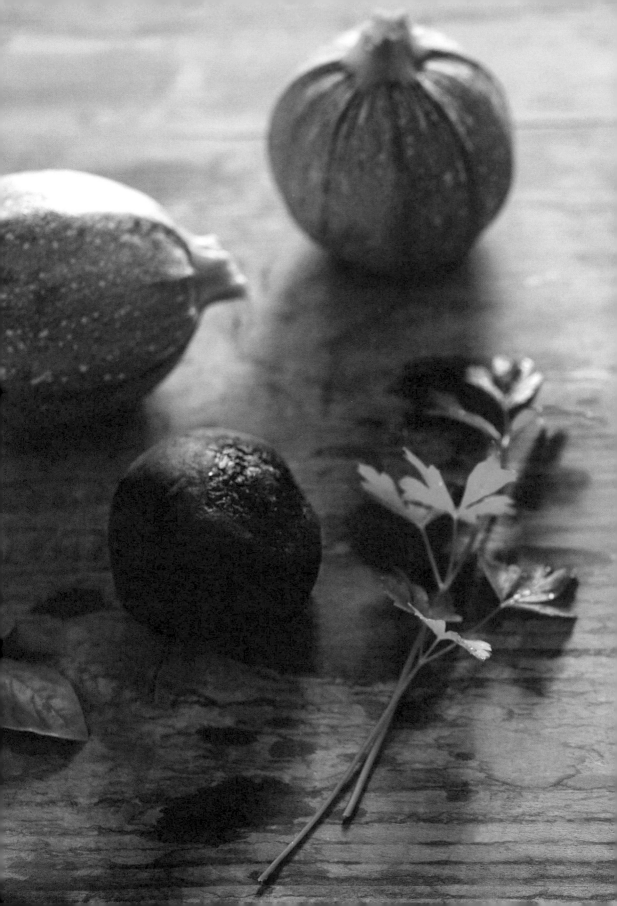

3

Principles of the Alkaline Cure

Guiding Principles of the Alkaline Cure
Be Mindful
How to Eat
What to Eat
When to Eat
How Much to Eat
Stay Hydrated
Exercise Regularly
Cleanse Your System
Enrich Your Surroundings
Find Your Rhythm

GUIDING PRINCIPLES OF THE ALKALINE CURE

The alkaline cure is a prescription for health, designed to help pull your body out of its acidic state by balancing your acid/alkaline intake. Remember, you do not need to cut out all acid foods; instead you should aim to eat fewer acid foods and more alkaline ones to redress a long-standing imbalance in your body's pH. You don't need to run a marathon; you need moderate and regular exercise. Your body doesn't want extremes, it wants balance.

It's important to pay attention to how you're eating and how you feel afterwards. Do you rush meals so you can move on to something else? Do you only chew a few times and then swallow food almost whole? Do you wash your food down with a drink during a meal? Do you eat on the run? All of these have a greater impact on your overall health than you may realise.

Eating alkaline means breaking away from some of the accepted norms that you may have grown accustomed to, particularly when it comes to portion size. Eating heavy acidic meals late at night really does harm your health. Paying attention to the quality of food you eat and having smaller portions should become your new norm. Choose fresh, local and seasonal products and combine them in the 2:1 ratio of alkaline to acidic foods.

The Alkaline Life

To reap the long-term benefits of this programme, we want to encourage you not only to think about the fourteen-day diet plan. This book should serve as a starting point for how to live alkaline. It introduces you to the ten principles preached and practised at The Original F. X. Mayr Health Center that will help guide you to healthy habits for life.

The first and most important principle is that of mindfulness, or what is sometimes called consciousness. The last principle echoes that philosophy by reminding us to find for ourselves the same regularity and rhythm in life that we can find in nature. This is the way to harmony and balance, not just in nutrition but in life.

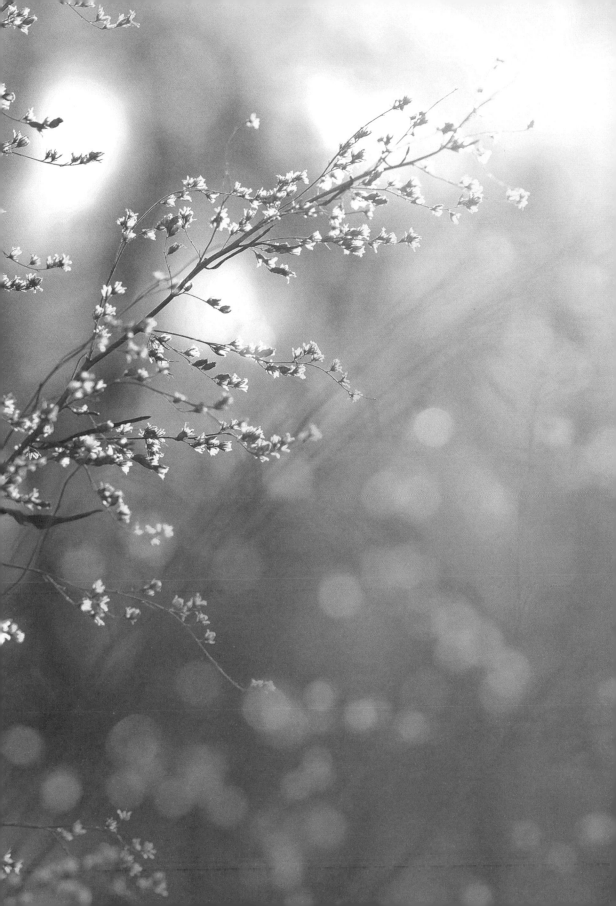

1. BE MINDFUL

Achieving long-term contentment, relaxation and general mental health is important if you want to lead a good-quality life. Stress, poor sleep and general unhappiness not only affect your day-to-day life, but they make your body more susceptible to illness and disease.

Balancing your body and your mind should start with awareness of how your body feels, how you respond emotionally to situations and your eating and lifestyle habits. It is about centering yourself, knowing yourself and being in calm control of yourself. There are techniques to help you develop good habits and a balanced lifestyle.

One method for balancing mind and body is MBSR (Mindfulness-Based Stress Reduction), a technique that helps prevent and treat burnout and stress-related illnesses. MBSR combines Buddhist meditation techniques and elements from yoga in a non-religious/non-esoteric way in order to train the mind. The aim is to make awareness part of your daily routine. This involves the conscious focus of attention to the moment with non-judgemental awareness and perception of your body, emotions and environment. This heightened awareness should enable you to observe these things more clearly and realistically and regulate your emotions.

The Benefits of Mindful Eating

Many of us have come to view meals as a necessity that can be rushed through to make time for doing other things, such as work, domestic chores or watching television. We regularly take meals on the run or at an office desk, and sometimes we even gulp down a plate of food at home. We move into autopilot and mechanically stab, chew and swallow. Even with healthy food, if we shovel it down quickly it doesn't get digested properly and stresses our systems. Mealtimes should be your own time, family time, a chance to anchor and be at one with the world. Considering how important food is to keeping us alive, we should give it more of our time. When we don't do that, we diminish our spirit, our nutrition. You won't always have time to do this, but erring towards this as often as possible is highly beneficial.

TEN STEPS FOR MINDFUL EATING

1. Give yourself time to eat. Allow at least thirty minutes at the table for each meal.

2. Make sure you are comfortably seated. Take a couple of deep breaths to settle yourself and accept that this is time set aside for a meal. Be thankful that you have nutritious food to eat.

3. Notice any feelings of impatience and urges to get on and just eat the food. Perhaps you are thinking of things you need to do, but try to concentrate. This time is dedicated to enjoying your food.

4. Look at the food on your plate. Appreciate its visual qualities. Smell your food. Breathe in the mouthwatering aromas.

5. Before you start to eat, think about how much food you put on your fork – the less, the better.

6. When you put the food in your mouth, take your time while chewing to appreciate the different flavours and textures.

7. Chew well, around thirty times is the minimum. Ensure the food in your mouth is fully masticated before you swallow.

8. Put your fork down between bites, it's important to take your time and rest so that you don't overwhelm your stomach.

9. Resist any urge to rush – perhaps on to dessert, to the next bite of food or to get up and do something else.

10. When you have finished, stay seated and relaxed for a few minutes. You should feel calm, satisfied and nourished, not bloated or overfull. Your body and your mind will thank you for taking extra time.

2. HOW TO EAT

The first law of eating well is to take your time. Do not eat when you are stressed or angry, which might cause you to hurry. When you do eat, it's important to set aside enough time to give your body a chance to absorb what it is being fed, especially at breakfast and lunch. You need to relearn the pleasures of eating properly.

Your body digests different foods in different parts of the digestive tract and needs time to carry out this process. It should come as no surprise that your body performs this task more efficiently when you are relaxed.

The Art of Chewing

Digestion starts in the mouth. Grinding food into smaller, softer pieces helps the gut to process it better. If your food isn't chewed well enough, you may end up feeling bloated and flatulent, as large pieces of food that pass through the stomach to the intestine attract more bacteria, which can generate gas and discomfort.

Nutrient absorption is also impaired by insufficient chewing and inefficient digestion. Chewing triggers the production of acids in the stomach, which break down the food so it can be absorbed. If you don't chew properly, other parts of the digestive system have to work harder to process the food, potentially making you feel lethargic.

Studies have shown that people who eat slowly tend to eat less and are, therefore, less likely to be overweight. The longer you take to chew your food, the longer you will take to finish your meal. As you eat, a message is sent to the brain to indicate you are getting full. If you eat too fast, the brain will think you are still hungry, even though you have consumed enough calories. Rushing through a meal may also prevent you from really tasting your food, leading to you not feeling satisfied by it. By taking your time, you have a chance to enjoy the unique flavours, textures and colours of the foods on your plate.

Chewing your food properly – as many as fifty times, according to Dr Mayr – not only breaks down your food into digestible pieces and better satisfies your appetite, but also brings your saliva into play.

An Exercise in Appreciating Food

The point of this eating exercise, which we practise at the clinic, is to show how something as humble as a raisin or sultana can teach us how to eat mindfully.

Take a raisin. Look at it carefully and smell it. Sense the sweet smell spreading through your nose, filling you with expectations of the taste. Put the raisin in your mouth and feel it with your tongue. Now chew carefully: notice how the taste spreads through your mouth. Observe how you feel and decide when you're ready to swallow. All the energy of the sun and the nutrients from the earth collected in that little raisin are in you now. You will digest it perfectly. This exercise should take about four minutes.

It is crucial that food spends sufficient time in the mouth to allow it to mix properly with saliva, an important digestive juice. A healthy person produces three to six cups of saliva per day. With some foods, chewing fifty times a mouthful can be difficult to achieve, but the process of mastication is beneficial, even if you are eating a lettuce leaf, because the saliva that chewing induces prepares the rest of the digestive system for the arrival of food.

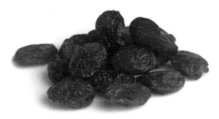

3. WHAT TO EAT

What you eat directly affects your alkaline/acid balance. As we mentioned earlier, the ideal alkaline to acid ratio is 2:1 – meaning every portion of acidic food on your plate should be paired with twice the amount of alkaline food.

However, it's not just the type of food that you eat but also the quality of your food that has a significant impact on your health. The mineral profiles of vegetables are affected by factors such as the soil they are grown in, since that is where the vegetables themselves source their nutrition. Therefore, we encourage you to look for fresh, seasonal, local foods of the best quality to make sure that what you eat is worthwhile both gastronomically and nutritionally. Organic produce is generally better because if your food is grown using pesticides and fertilisers, it may be nutritionally depleted.

Eat From the Land Around You
Food always has a greater nutritional value when it comes from the land and sea near your home. The greater the distance it has travelled, the more hands will have touched it, and the more likely it will have been processed or acidified along the way. In addition to having greater freshness and quality, locally produced food is often sourced from smaller craft businesses that contribute to your local economy. Generally, the larger the business, especially in the food industry, the larger the quality compromises that have been made.

Pick Food for Each Season
Foods at optimum ripeness contain the maximum amount of nutrients. This is especially true of fruit. Our lives are rhythmical and we should follow the changes as they happen. Supermarkets tend to make us believe there is only one season, where everything is available all the time. This is a myth. Depending on where you live, strawberries may be ripe in July, plums in September, apples in October, beetroot in November. In markets and small shops it's easier to buy one or two vegetables at a time to get a good variety. Multipacks of fruit and vegetables tend to fill the refrigerator and may not get used until they are past their best.

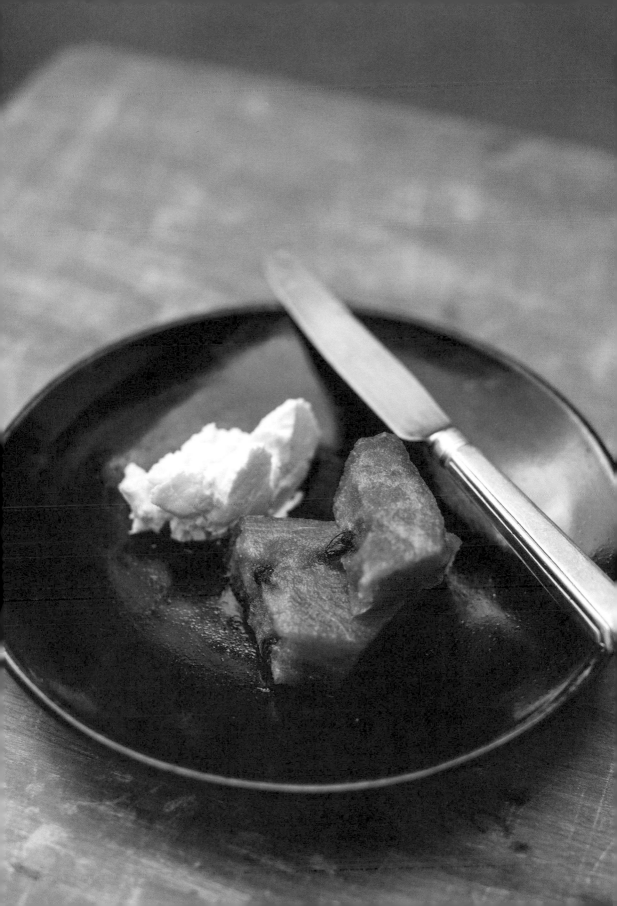

4. WHEN TO EAT

Make the most important meals of the day breakfast and lunch. When you wake in the morning your body is at its most able, in a digestive sense. It can cope with a wide range of different foods more easily. But in the evening, your body, like your mind, is slowing down, so you need to eat smaller portions of more easily digested foods. The habit of eating substantial meals later in the evening is not good from a digestive point of a view. Evening meals should be consumed early, preferably before six in the evening, since eating late can have several effects including:

* **Sleep deprivation:** Your body's rhythms are programmed to complete the digestive process within twenty-four hours. Eating late disrupts this rhythm. Your body starts to slow down after sunset, preparing for sleep at nightfall. During sleep, your body and your digestive system need a break to cleanse and prepare for the next day. If you eat a meal as your body is winding down in the evening, then your metabolism is forced to gear up to digest the food, using energy while you sleep. This activity can result in poor sleep and lethargy.

* **Acid reflux:** When you eat a meal and then lie down to sleep, your horizontal position may allow acid from your stomach to travel up the oesophagus, which can cause inflammation and heartburn.

Raw Only Before Four

Raw foods are highly nutritious but they are also more difficult to digest. In their uncooked forms, they take longer for your body to break down. If you eat raw food in the evening and then go to sleep, the chances are that these foods will not be digested properly and will hang around in the gut while you sleep. Far from being refreshed, your stomach wakes up to a new job – sorting out last night's dinner. By all means eat raw foods earlier in the day, but make sure your body has enough time to deal with them before you go to bed.

5. HOW MUCH TO EAT

Most of us eat too much – more than we need, more than our bodies
are designed to cope with and more than our bodies need nutritionally.
If your diet is varied enough to include a complete spectrum of
vitamins, minerals and amino acids, then you don't actually have to
eat that much. Yet many of us do. This is especially true of meat. The
definition of 'too much' is different for different people, which is why
in Mayr therapy treatment plans are always personalised.

Given the strong likelihood that for many years the balance of
your diet may have been skewed towards acid foods (see page 68), we
suggest eating increased amounts of alkaline foods to compensate.
Aim for a ratio of 4:1 (alkaline:acid) for a few weeks to boost the
cleansing process.

The stomach can take up to four hours to process a meal. It's
therefore important to leave enough time before eating again. It's not
wise to dump fresh food on top of part-digested food. The stomach
needs to deal with one load at a time and adjust its acidity accordingly.

Drink water, vegetable tea or herbal tea between meals, but avoid
drinking while you are eating.

Portion Control Made Easy

If you fill your stomach with too much food, you will stretch and
overwhelm it. It's common to eat meals that are two, three or
sometimes four times larger than our stomachs. That's not what we
are designed to do.

If you do this, your body has to pump more and more energy into
digesting the unusually large load. This leads to exhaustion of your
body's systems, leaving you physically and mentally lacking in energy.
Overeating is also wasteful and inefficient – your body can only absorb
only a limited amount nutrients before your food is excreted. If you eat
too much, a lot of the food will just be turned to waste.

Reducing portion size is an easy way to limit your intake. At the
clinic we recommend eating off smaller plates, and using a small spoon
rather than a large one to provide a visual explanation of what we are
trying to achieve. Make every mouthful count and enjoy eating.

6. STAY HYDRATED

Water is one of the most important aspects of an alkaline diet. It helps clean the body and keeps us hydrated. This obviously requires us to start drinking it early in the morning and also develop a taste and respect for it. Drinking water helps circulate nutrients around the body and flushes out toxins. Keeping hydrated is also particularly good for the skin. Given how important it is, it is worth taking more seriously.

The more liquid you can consume, the more it will help to cleanse the body. You should drink at least two litres of water a day (if you weigh around 68 kilograms, more if you are heavier). Plain water is the best option, but tisanes, herbal teas and vegetable teas can be counted as part of your intake.

However, drinking while eating is not good because it dilutes your valuable saliva and stomach acid. Drink half an hour before or after meals. If you have water at the table, the temptation is to wash your food down your throat. Not only will that dilute the saliva and deprive your stomach of an important stimulus, but it also creates a distraction to the main event, digesting food. Water is valuable but not at the same time as food. There is drinking time and there is eating time.

A Note on Alkaline Water

Alkaline, or ionised, water is water that has a pH reading above 7. Like alkaline foods, alkaline water can be used to counteract the effects of an over-acidic diet. Water can be alkalised by using an ionising unit, but two much simpler methods to improve your water's alkalinity are either to add a little bicarbonate of soda or squeeze a few drops of lemon or lime into a glass of warm water. Both lemon and lime, although acidic, are in fact alkaline-forming.

THE WORLD OF WATER

Pure Water
Pure water is clean, filtered water free from bacteria. It is not mineral-rich and serves to cleanse the body, rather than enrich it. It should have a pH value of 7 and, as such, is neutral. You may assume that all water is neutral in pH but this is not the case, as you will read.

Bottled and Mineral Water
Good minerals in water are especially valuable because we digest them more easily when we drink them rather than eat them. Bottled mineral waters vary widely between very alkaline and mildly alkaline. Often the pH of bottled mineral water will be listed on the label, but you can easily check for yourself with a pH strip.

Popular brands vary a lot in the levels of minerals they contain. Bicarbonates are alkalising, so together with dissolved solids such as calcium and magnesium, they can create a beneficial effect that will restore nutrients directly to bones, which may have become weakened as a result of countering acid attacks.

You need fewer minerals in the morning, because you really just want to flush the system. However, in the afternoon, mineral water is an ideal way of delivering minerals to your body.

Distilled Water
Distilled water, while exceptionally pure and free of impurities, is known as 'dead water', because it has lost the ability to polarise light and thus, it has no energetic value for the cells.

Tap Water
Tap water is more likely to be acidic than alkaline, and while that is not a significant issue because the acidity is low, you can nevertheless alkalise it. However, be aware that tap water often contains unwanted chemicals (e.g. chlorine, fluoride, pesticides, etc.) or heavy metals (e.g. aluminium, lead, etc.) so it is advisable to filter it.

7. EXERCISE REGULARLY

Exercise aids weight loss, strengthens muscles (which support your skeletal system), improves blood flow and stimulates the brain to produce dopamine – a hormone known to lift mood.

The stronger you are physically, the better you support your digestive system. For instance, core fitness supports the intestinal system. Regular exercise does not have to be strenuous to be beneficial. Walking is a natural motion; running long distances perhaps less so. Body movements that shift your frame, your stomach and your chest are a part of keeping supple and toned. You should aim for a minimum of thirty minutes of deliberate cardio exercise every day – walk or cycle to work, or take the stairs instead of the lift. Some simple stretching exercises are good, too. For long walks, use walking sticks – the ones used for alpine walking – because they open up the chest, exercise the top half of the torso and prevent you from hunching.

Be Gentle with Your Body

Be realistic and mindful of your current health status. Exercise in moderation. This not a competition; it is about you and making you feel better. Excessive exercise can be acid-forming. Short, sharp bursts of exercise are fine occasionally if you enjoy them, but they are not strictly necessary. A regular routine of steady body movement will deliver the results you need. Routine is the key word here, but to avoid monotony, try a variety of forms of exercise that involve different parts of the body.

Find Your Naturally Healthy Shape

The point of exercise is to keep the body functioning through its natural easy rhythms that support our natural shape. If you adopt a sedentary lifestyle, your body shape can change and your internal organs may struggle to operate freely. Damaging habits include driving for long distances hunched over the steering wheel or bending over a keyboard for long periods. You need to take exercise that stretches your body back into place. Many types of exercise are beneficial. Consider trying a dance class to kick start your cure.

8. CLEANSE YOUR SYSTEM

Dr Mayr worked for many years at the Carlsbad spa. There he learned the therapeutic value of the highly mineralised Carlsbad waters. Today, at The Original F. X. Mayr Health Center, we use Epsom salts as a purgative: one level tablespoon to 235 millilitres of warm water taken in the morning on an empty stomach. It is important to note that we do not recommend you do this kind of intestinal cleanse at home without supervision.

The scientific name for Epsom salts is magnesium sulphate, and it is the same highly mineralised salt that is used in agriculture to put magnesium (an essential element of chlorophyll found in plants) back into the soil.

The effect is to put internal pressure on the intestinal tract and to stimulate the liver and gall bladder by promoting the release of bile from the gall bladder, which makes the liver produce new bile. This cleans out any toxins that may have built up over time and encourages the intestine to work effectively.

At the clinic, we also use what we call base powder, which is essentially bicarbonate of soda or baking soda. We may also add minerals such as calcium and potassium. The effect is to immediately alkalise the stomach and trigger the movement of food through the digestive system. We recommend taking a base powder mixed in water or warm milk on a regular basis.

Give Your Stomach a Rest

Allowing your body time to recuperate is an important part of our programme, and the first week of the alkaline cure is designed to give your digestive system a rest. Rest for the stomach means reducing the amount you eat, eating nutritionally beneficial foods and simplifying the combinations of foods you eat so they are easy to digest. Resting the stomach may also involve simple fasting where you consume only tea or water so as not to stress the stomach.

After the stomach has rested, you can begin to eat meals in which different ingredients and recipes are gradually introduced.

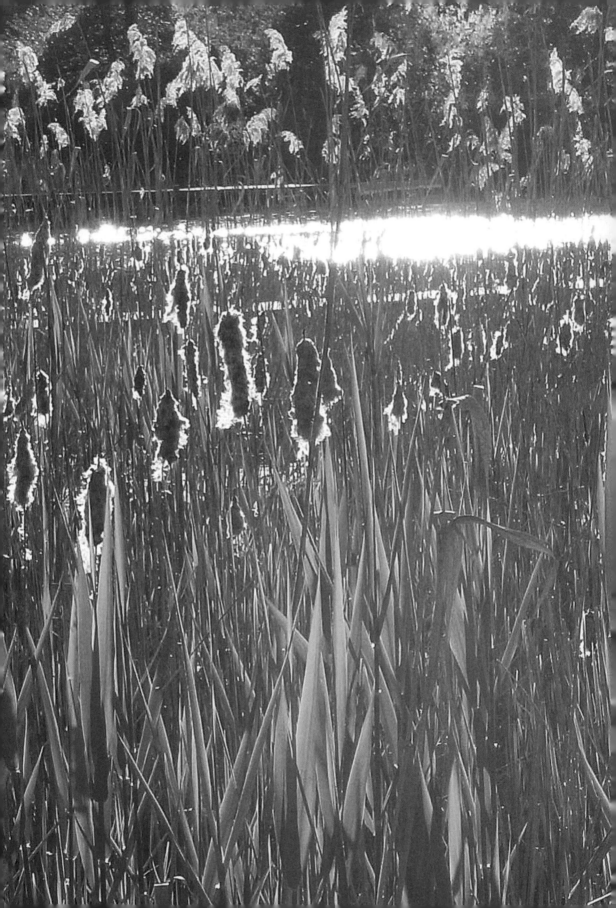

9. ENRICH YOUR SURROUNDINGS

At our clinic we enjoy the wonderful forest and mountains around us. The lake where the clinic is situated, Lake Wörthersee, is unusual in that it is a well-used recreational lake, but the waters are still clean enough to drink. We are fortunate to have hot summers and snowy winters and we can enjoy the changing seasons and the fresh air throughout the year. At times we may take our environment for granted, but not everyone is so lucky.

How we live is also a reminder of how we set out to cleanse and improve our inner health. It's worth acquiring a few simple items for the home: candles that provide a soft light, calming music to look forward to, and a new water jug and glass, to make your increased fluid intake a treat. Simple things such as these can help mark your progress.

Create a Healthy Home Environment
Your home environment has a significant impact on your health and well-being. Even if you live in an inner-city flat, making a few changes to your home can bring enormous benefits:

* Buy some fresh flowers and plants for each room. They are a reminder of nature, remove toxins from the air and produce oxygen. Research shows that adding plants to hospital rooms helped to speed recovery rates of patients who have had surgery.

* Open the windows to improve air flow.

* Switch to a less toxic range of household cleaning products. Many cleaning products contain volatile compounds that we may inhale, exposing us to chemicals and toxins. Some of these may mimic oestrogen and can interfere with our hormones.

* Play pleasurable music – either to energise or relax you.

* Turn off computers and electrical devices in the bedrooms when not in use, but especially when you are asleep. Appliance lights can stimulate your senses and prevent full, deep sleep. Some experts also believe that overexposure to the radiation from electrical devices can adversely affect your health.

10. FIND YOUR RHYTHM

Life is governed by rhythms and cycles. Day. Night. Summer. Winter. Our bodies respond to these natural cycles. Sometimes we have to remind ourselves that these changes are good – even a harsh winter after summer purges the ground as well as our souls. We work hard, we rest, we sleep, we are renewed and we start again. These rhythms and cycles are essential to our well-being and distinguish us from machines.

We are not machines but we sometimes drive ourselves as if we were. Of course it is admirable to work long hours, to push yourself and to achieve. But once you have achieved what you set out to do, it's essential to allow your body time to recuperate. Try to find the off switch and turn off the engine. It is not lazy to break off and take time out. It is necessary.

Settle and Restore

If you eat on the run or if you squeeze meals between other activities, you are overruling your body's natural instinct to rest and restore. You are putting it under stress. If necessary, you need to reinvent these restorative rhythms and create breaks throughout the day.

When you go on holiday, you can immediately feel the benefit of change. Your everyday world recedes and you cease to worry so much about the things that seemed so important last week. You get some sunshine and your mood improves. The body also feels better and is better able to release acids naturally in a hot and sunny climate. In winter it tends to want to cling on to them in case it might need them. During the cold months it is fine to find energy in hot foods like porridge, but in the summer your body wants salads and fruits. Follow your seasonal instincts.

Equally, if you are one of those people who does not like to eat breakfast early in the morning, that is not a problem – eat a bit later when you are ready. Adjust your routine to suit you. If you are happy on two meals a day, that is fine. If you feel you need four meals, that's all right too – just make them smaller. Take control of your routine and your body will be grateful.

Your Body's Thermostat

Your body regulates its own temperature for
different times of the day. At night, it cools internally
in preparation for sleep, which is why a hot bath helps
muscles relax – a hot external environment causes the body
to cool down inside. For daily activity, the body needs to
be warmer, which is why a cool shower in the morning
raises your internal temperature and primes your body
for the day ahead.

Rhythm and Routine

Routines structure the day and will give you back a sense of purpose.
Drink a glass of warm water when you wake up. Start the day with
an exfoliating skin brush (see page 98) and morning shower. Open
the windows and try some stretching exercises. Go for a short walk
to breathe the air outside and then have breakfast.

Rest and Recuperation

With the increasing speed and intensity of modern living, rest is as
important as work – even a nap in the afternoon can be a good thing.
You must realise that you cannot keep doing everything at the same
fast pace. Try to interrupt your working routine every ninety minutes
or so. Ideally, you should operate on ninety-minute cycles: seventy-five
minutes of concentration and fifteen minutes of rest and recuperation.
Rest time should be a deliberate break. Open a window or go for a
stroll. And be sure to make time for lunch – thirty minutes' eating time
at least. Remember to vary your restorative activities. Have a water
break in the afternoon. If you get tired later in the day, it may well be
due to the foods you ate at lunch and which were probably eaten too
quickly. If you're in a hurry, don't gulp down food. It's much better to
wait until you have more time to eat.

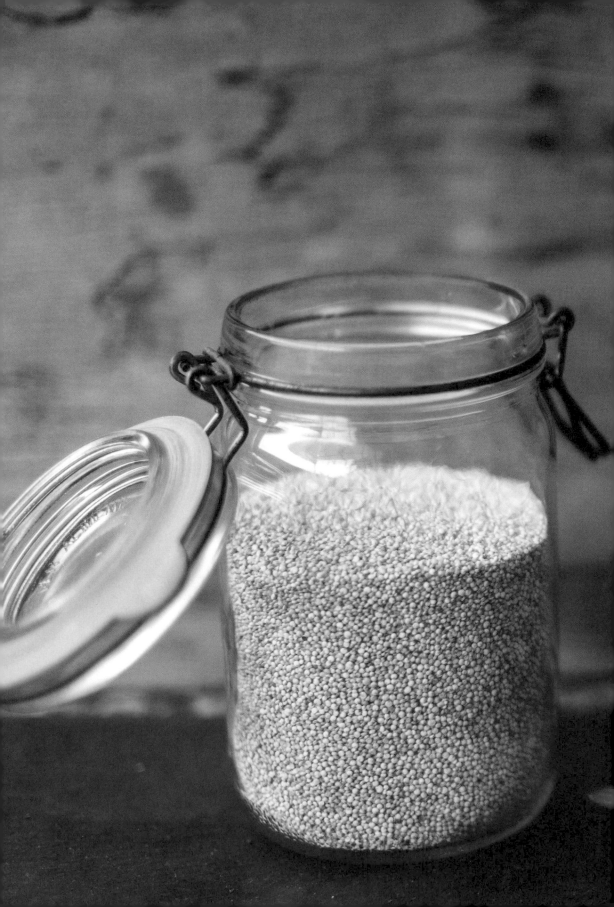

4

Preparing To
Go Alkaline

An Alkaline Way of Life
Acid Food Groups
Alkaline Food Groups
20 Alkaline Superfoods
The Alkaline Kitchen

AN ALKALINE WAY OF LIFE

Before starting the alkaline cure, it's important to understand the different foods around you and their impact on your body. By understanding the associated benefits and harmful effects of alkaline and acidic foods, you will have the knowledge you need to shop and fill your store cupboard more conscientiously. Once you've set up your alkaline kitchen and are familiar with the foods, tools and cooking methods, you can then start on the quick and easy road to an alkaline way of life.

HOW THE BODY USES FOOD

Food contains nutrients that provide our body with energy and help control growth. There are six main groups of nutrients that the body needs: water, carbohydrates, protein, fats, minerals and vitamins.

Water: The Holy Grail of Health
We can live without the other five nutrients for weeks, but we can survive only a few days without water. It forms the basis of our blood, digestive juices, urine and perspiration. Water's functions include regulating body temperature through sweating, maintaining the health and integrity cells, lubricating joints, carrying nutrients and oxygen to cells, and moisturising skin to maintain its texture and appearance.

Carbohydrates: Fast and Slow Release Energy
Your body uses carbohydrates to make glucose for energy. Carbohydrates are found in fruit, vegetables, grains, milk and any food that contains sugar. Carbohydrates are split into two categories, simple and complex. Sugar is a simple carbohydrate, meaning your body metabolises it straight away for energy.

Starches are complex carbohydrates. Starch-rich foods, such as beans and grains, release energy more slowly, as your body has to break the starch down into sugar before it can use it. Fibre, which is the indigestible material present in many complex carbohydrates, serves to accelerate the movement of food through the system and affects how nutrients are absorbed.

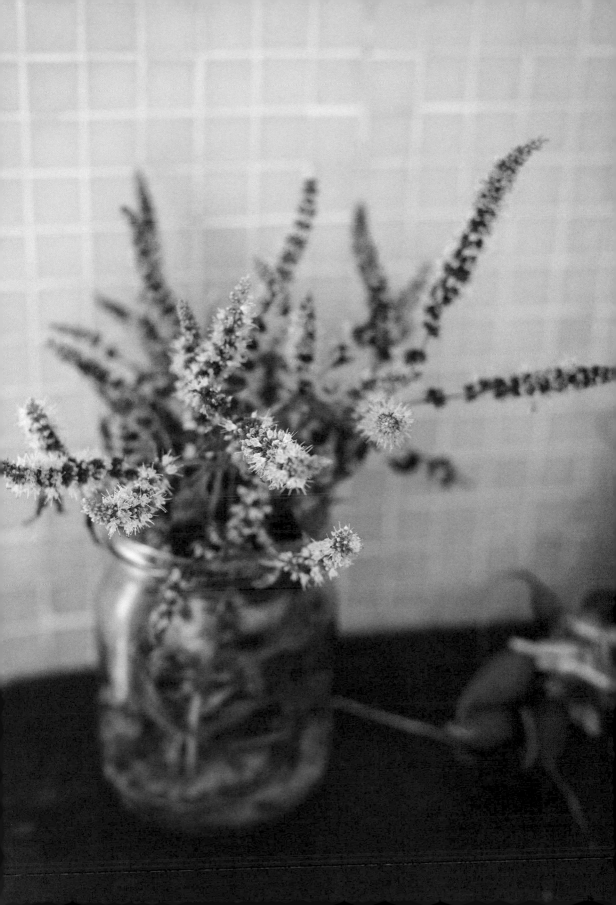

Protein: The Building Blocks of DNA

All foods contain protein, but in varying amounts. Protein is made up of chains of amino acids – the building blocks of DNA. Your body needs nine essential amino acids from your diet since it cannot synthesise these for itself. A complete protein is a single food source that contains the nine amino acids in the correct proportions. There are not many complete protein foods, which is why you need to eat a varied diet to gain all the essential amino acids.

Fats and Oils: The Good, the Bad and the Ugly

Fats are essential for energy, proper brain and nerve function, healthy skin and transporting the fat-soluble vitamins A, D, E and K.

There are various categories of fat, with unsaturated being the healthiest, followed by the unhealthier saturated and finally the unhealthiest – trans fats. Unsaturated fats are mostly found in plant-based foods such as nuts, seeds, vegetable and seed oils, and oily fish, as well as peanuts and avocados. Saturated fats are found mostly in animal products: meat, cheese, milk, butter and eggs. Trans fats can be natural or artificial, but are mostly created through hydrogenation, a process that is used in the production of fast foods, fried foods and mass-produced baked products.

Minerals: Strong Bones and Healthy Blood

Minerals are inorganic nutrients that perform a variety of functions in the body. Calcium and magnesium, for example, are important for remineralising bones and teeth. Iron is a component of haemoglobin, which carries oxygen in red blood cells. The best mineral and vitamin sources include vegetables, fruits and foods derived from animals.

Vitamins: The Full Spectrum

The body needs a variety of vitamins to stay healthy. Vitamin A helps skin and hair grow; vitamin C helps fight infections; and vitamin D, synthesised by the skin using sunlight, aids the formation of teeth and bones.

ACID FOOD GROUPS

The foods below are categorised by the strength of their acidity. Remember, rather than cutting out all acid foods, we advise that you reduce your consumption of acid foods and replace them by introducing more alkaline foods into your diet.

Strongly Acid-forming Foods

Animal protein: pork, fish, chicken, lamb, beef

*

Aged dairy products: matured cheese

*

Refined oils and fats: margarine, corn oil

*

Industrially processed products, canned foods

*

Foods containing refined sugar and
flour: preserves, fizzy drinks, cakes, sweets,
chocolate, white bread

*

Coffee, alcohol

Mildly Acid-forming Foods

Vegetable protein: chickpeas, beans, lentils

*

Fresh dairy products: fresh cheese

*

Nuts: cashews, peanuts, pistachios

ACID-FORMING FOODS

Animal Protein and Fish

During the digestion of foods with sulphur-containing amino acids, such as animal proteins, our bodies produce sulphuric acid as a by-product. So all meat is acidic, almost by definition, although lean cuts tend to be less acidic than fattier parts, and fresh meats less acidic than processed meats, which contain a lot of additives and preservatives. For these reasons we advise that you eat meat only on alternate days.

Fish is another source of protein that is not alkaline. It can offer nutritional benefits such as omega-3 essential fatty acids and complements alkaline vegetables, such as leeks, spinach, potatoes and red peppers, so we could term fish 'alkaline friendly' for that reason.

Milk and Dairy

Fresh milk and fresh (non-aged) cheese can feature in an alkaline diet, although they are slightly acidic as they consist primarily of animal protein and fat. Dr Mayr was a great advocate of milk as a nutritious food but the milk he recommended was unpasteurised and from organic farms near the clinic. Pasteurisation has become standard but the process of heating depletes milk of much of its nutritional value. When it comes to cheese, goat's milk cheese is easier to digest and better for those with allergies than cow's milk cheese.

A Note on Curd Cheese

Curd cheese is similar to quark and cottage cheese. It is a by-product of souring milk with rennet or lemon to separate curds and whey. If you cannot find it locally, you can make your own by draining cottage cheese through muslin and then mashing it. As an alternative, you can also use thick, probiotic yogurt.

Vegetable Protein

Many vegetable proteins are mildly acidic, such as chickpeas, lentils, some soy products and certain types of beans, but they have the advantage over animal proteins of not containing saturated fat.

Bread

The yeast in bread tends to encourage acidic conditions in your body and may predispose you to candida infection. By avoiding yeast products, you may find yourself less bloated. Gluten reactions from wheat and rye tend to be more noticeable as we age, so focus on flatbreads, crispbreads or any breads that are made without yeast.

Refined Oils and Fats

Refined oils and fats tend to be higher in saturated and trans fats – the latter more dangerous than the former. Both raise levels of 'bad' (LDL) cholesterol, increasing the risk of heart disease, but trans fats also lower levels of 'good' (HDL) cholesterol and therefore can be considered more damaging.

Refined Sugar

There is enough natural sugar in our diet without supplementing it. While it's best to avoid adding sugar to food, if you need it, there are natural alternatives such as stevia, which is sweeter than cane sugar.

It's important to note that the sugar in whole fruit is better than sugar eaten on its own or in processed food since fruit contains fibre, which slows the absorption of sugar.

Caffeine and Alcohol

Caffeine is one of the most acidic ingredients you can consume. An occasional cup of freshly ground coffee is fine, but daily consumption of caffeine-containing drinks is known to leach minerals from bones to buffer the acidity caused by the caffeine.

Alcohol is as acidic as caffeine. Try to avoid drinking alcohol, but if you do want an occasional alcoholic drink, choose an additive- and preservative-free organic beer.

ALKALINE FOOD GROUPS

Nearly all vegetables, herbs, root spices (such as garlic and ginger), many fruits (provided they are ripe) and cold-pressed oils are alkaline. Some people are sensitive to certain vegetables, and if you feel they are not doing you any good, then simply avoid eating them.

Alkaline-forming Foods

Vegetables: broccoli, cabbage, spinach, kale,
salad leaves, potatoes, sweet potatoes, beansprouts,
beetroot, cucumber

*

Ripe fruits: bananas, watermelon, papaya, mango

*

Grains: amaranth, quinoa,
rye, buckwheat

*

Fresh, aromatic herbs: basil, rosemary, thyme

*

Nuts: almonds

*

High-quality, cold-pressed 'virgin'
vegetable, nut and seed oils: flaxseed oil, olive oil,
pumpkin seed oil, hempseed oil

*

Pure and mineral water, herbal teas,
vegetable teas

ALKALINE-FORMING FOODS

Vegetables have always been a crucial part of an alkaline diet. Not only are they nutritional powerhouses, but vegetables are delicious and often form a key part of the menu in top restaurants. In Paris, Alain Passard has three Michelin stars for his restaurant, L'Arpège, where each day one menu is dedicated to the produce from his garden. He offers dishes such as celery risotto with herb emulsion, celeriac mousseline with turnips and lemon, and root vegetables with couscous, argan oil and celery emulsion – all very alkaline.

An alkaline diet is a prescription for a healthier lifestyle and also healthier agriculture. Our taste buds instinctively prefer fresh and locally grown – or, even better, homegrown – vegetables because their nutritional value diminishes if they are left to linger in the back of a truck, on a supermarket shelf or, worse, in a warehouse.

It is never a question of either-or with vegetables. Cooking two, three or even four kinds of vegetables together brings a more complete nutritional spectrum to the dish and providing colour on the plate is always good.

Leafy Green Vegetables

Green and leafy vegetables, such as broccoli, sprouts, cabbage and spinach are more than just backdrops to the meal. They are high in vitamin A – essential for healthy skin, hair and nails – and vitamin C, a potent antioxidant. Kale and other leafy greens are a good source of iron and calcium. These vegetables are versatile in cooking, adding fresh and interesting flavours to dishes. The water in which a cauliflower is steamed also makes excellent stock for an alkaline vegetable tea. The leaves around a cauliflower are nutritious and tasty.

Salad leaves are more than just garnish, they're a valuable first course and a way of incorporating vegetable oil dressings (such as pumpkin oil, virgin olive oil and flaxseed oil), seeds, small fruits (such as cranberries and pomegranate seeds), and a generous handful of fresh herbs. All salad leaves are alkaline. Lettuce is surprisingly nutritious: two cups of romaine lettuce will give you more than enough vitamins A and K for the day. Iceberg is not quite as nutritious, but still contains vitamin B, potassium, manganese, iron, calcium and phosphorous.

A Note on Antioxidants

Antioxidants are nutrients and enzymes that help
fight the damaging effects of free radicals by neutralising
them. Free radicals are highly reactive chemicals that
damage our cells and are said to cause cancer. Alkalising
foods, such as strawberries, prunes, kale and spinach, are
packed with antioxidants including beta-carotene,
lycopene, and vitamins A, C and E.

It also contains a fair amount of copper and zinc. The zesty rocket is
a rich food in terms of minerals and vitamins. Any alkaline lunch can
start with a good salad.

Beansprouts

Sprouting beans and seeds are highly nutritious. Alfalfa is one of the
most commonly found, but many other pulses can be sprouted as well.
Sprouting boosts nutritional value, and beansprouts are often easier
than other vegetables for the body to digest. Sprouting is a fun and
easy kitchen activity that bears valuable results.

Roots and Tubers

Roots and tubers provide the framework for an alkaline diet – not just
potatoes but beetroot, carrots, celeriac, parsnips, radishes, swedes and
turnips can all provide the basis of an alkaline meal. Steamed, mashed
or baked, they submit happily to nearly every culinary innovation.
Some, such as carrot and celeriac, are also famously good just grated
into their own raw salad – the former with a few currants and an
orange dressing, the latter with a flaxseed mayonnaise.

Other Vegetables

All squashes, are alkaline, as are courgettes, cucumber and pumpkin.
The stem and stalk vegetables – such as globe artichokes, asparagus,

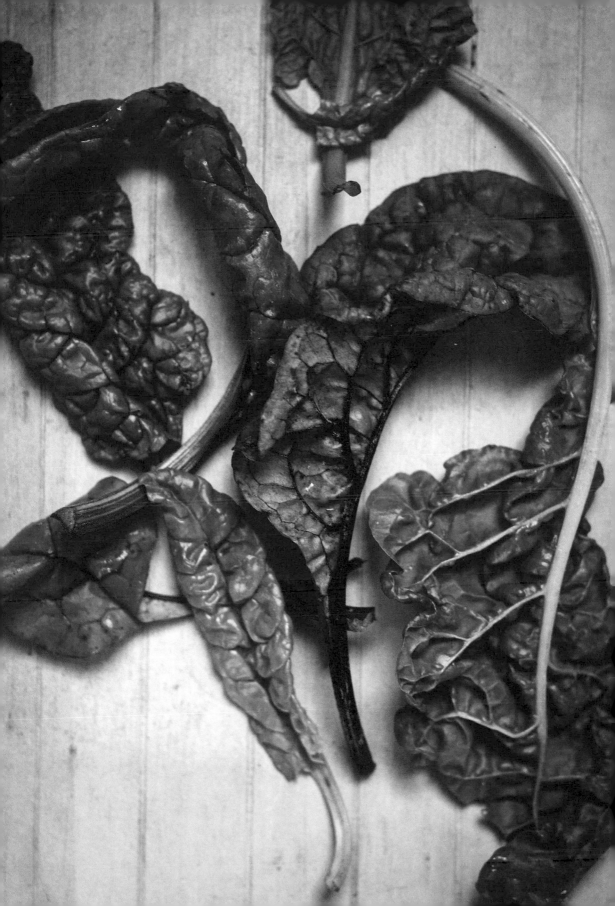

celery and fennel – again are all alkaline and packed with minerals, vitamins and fibre. A meal comprised of one vegetable from each of the above categories would be a feast indeed and nearly all can be puréed to bring other dimensions into your meals.

We tend to take onions and leeks for granted, but both are the base of many regional cuisines around the world and are an easy way to slip some fresh alkalising vitamins into your cooking.

FRUIT

The problem with fruit is that, very often, it is not ripe. If fruit has not had enough time to ripen naturally – or has been chemically ripened in storage – then it simply does not have the equivalent nutritional value.

A strawberry rushed around the globe to decorate a supermarket shelf will not have the same value as a strawberry freshly picked from a garden in its optimum season. Tomatoes, too, are classified as a fruit and need to be very ripe for maximum nutritional benefit. As bananas ripen, indicated by brown spots, the starch starts to turn to sugar, which provides excellent fast-acting energy for our cells.

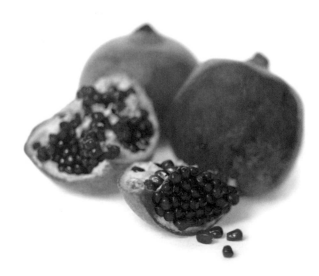

Melons are a wonderful alkaline fruit and can be easily digested because they are mostly water, which enables the body to absorb their nutrients quickly and easily. Watermelon is one of the most alkaline of all fruits.

Dried Fruit

Drying fruits can be an effective way of preserving the alkalinity, especially in the case of ripe fruits, provided they have not been dipped in a solution of ascorbic acid, citric acid, sodium metabisulphite or sugar, which can all undermine the fruit's alkalinity. Read the labels. Properly and naturally dried, fruits such as currants, apricots, mangoes, plums and bananas can be welcome alkaline additions to snacks, breakfasts and salads. The low temperatures of drying in the oven or in a specialist food dehydrator help retain nutrients that cooking might otherwise destroy.

Dried fruits can form an important source of fibre, which can help ease constipation. They are also a good source of potassium, vitamins and minerals – for example, apricots and peaches contain vitamin A for skin support, figs contain calcium for bone health, and plums contain vitamin K, another nutrient that helps bone development.

If you are drying fruit at home, use lemon as a preservative, which boosts the alkalising effect and prevents discolouration. Drying can be a lengthy process: thin apple slices will take about six hours in an oven at 60°C and peach halves may take up to thirty-six hours.

GRAINS

Grains are incredibly versatile and nutritious. They have been cultivated and used in various forms for much of human history. But wheat, the most popular grain, is now so widely cultivated, modified and processed that by the time it turns up in supermarkets as bagels and sliced white bread, it has often lost most of its nutritional value.

Commercially, wheat tends to top everything else in terms of being fast-growing, high-yielding and hardier than other crops. But it is only when we look at the health benefits of other grains that we can see how other crops offer greater nutritional depth and health benefits.

A Note on Gluten

Awareness of gluten intolerance has increased in
recent years. At the clinic we test all our patients.
Sometimes, eating less gluten is enough to avoid an allergic
reaction, but if you have a gluten allergy, you may have
to stick to eating gluten-free grains, such as millet, or
pseudocereals, such as amaranth,
quinoa and buckwheat.

A World of Grains
The traditional foods of other cultures provide many examples of the
wide variety of nutritious grains available. Rye contains more amino
acids, fibre and vitamin E than wheat, and it also has a lower gluten
content. Amaranth and quinoa are high in fibre as well as the essential
amino acid lysine, which helps build muscle and tissue, and boosts the
nutritional impact of the protein sources it is paired with. Buckwheat
is also a source of lysine, and buckwheat noodles – known as soba
noodles in Japan – are a healthy alternative to white pasta.

Amaranth, quinoa and buckwheat, though they can be used and
eaten like other cereals, are actually pseudocereals. True cereals, such as
wheat, oats and rice, are derived from grasses, while pseudocereals are
derived from other kinds of plants. Pseudocereals often have a more
complex nutritional profile and do not contain gluten.

Mixing different grains is, in itself, a good dietary practice because
each has its own attributes and contains a cocktail of amino acids.
Adding healthy grains to traditional breakfast dishes such as porridge
and granola is an easy way to gain additional nutritional benefits from
those meals.

THE POWER OF HERBS AND SPICES

Herbs and spices are as universally alkaline as meat is universally acid. They also bring other benefits in terms of minerals and vitamins. The aim is to bring them into our diet more readily so they can start to play a more fundamental role.

Herbs

Parsley is a simple, versatile herb; use it generously. It is rich in antioxidants, potassium, calcium, manganese, iron and magnesium. There are more than thirty varieties, all of which taste markedly different. At one extreme, we have the tightly furled, curly variety and, at the other, the fragrant flat leaf.

Every sprig has two uses: the stalks help make flavoursome stocks and can be added directly into soups – use string to hold them together so they can be taken out later. The leaves can be added at the end of the cooking to add some colour and freshness.

Other herbs such as basil, rosemary, thyme, sage, marjoram and chervil all make wonderful additions to meals and bring with them many health benefits as well. These small but potent leaves are packed with everything from antioxidants, potassium, iron and calcium to manganese, magnesium and selenium. Plus they provide the body with B-complex vitamins, beta-carotene, folic acid and vitamins A, K, E and C. These herbs are known to fight cancer, boost brain function, aid digestion, increase circulation and have anti-inflammatory and antiviral properties.

Root Herbs

Garlic and ginger are some of the more powerful members of the root family. Ginger makes a potent tea. Garlic tea is often recommended for candida. Four peeled and crushed cloves should be steeped for twenty minutes in 950 millilitres of hot water with a grating of ginger and a few drops of lemon. Horseradish has been used for centuries to treat a variety of ailments, from urinary tract infection to gout. Horseradish can be shaved and mixed with lemon and a little curd. Just a few gratings of the fresh root can dramatically change the taste of a dish. It goes especially well with beetroot.

A Note on Candida

Candida, a type of yeast, is the most common cause
of fungal infection in humans, and it thrives in acidic
environments. When candida levels get out of control, they
can cause a host of health problems, including the yeast
infection commonly known as thrush, bloating and severe
allergic reactions. The best way to treat candida is by healing
the gut: eliminating sugar, fermented foods and alcohol
(all of which candida feeds off), reducing carbohydrate
intake and eating foods that fight candida, such as garlic,
ginger and parsley.

Seeds and Spices

Although small, seeds deliver a disproportionately high nutritional
value into the diet. Seeds need to be freshly ground using a grinder or
a pestle and mortar and, once ground, will not keep at their best for
more than a few hours. Flaxseed (linseed), sunflower seeds, pine nuts,
pumpkin seeds, sesame seeds and wheatgerm are all good alkaline
companions to sprinkle on salads or on porridge. Seeds can also be
sprouted, in the same way as alfalfa.

Spices are derived from seeds. Experiment with new spice mixes,
such as coriander and fennel seeds, which can be scattered on cooked
dishes. Or put spices in a pepper mill on the table for everyone else
to help themselves. Spices are a quick way to perk up your food, both
taste-wise and nutritionally.

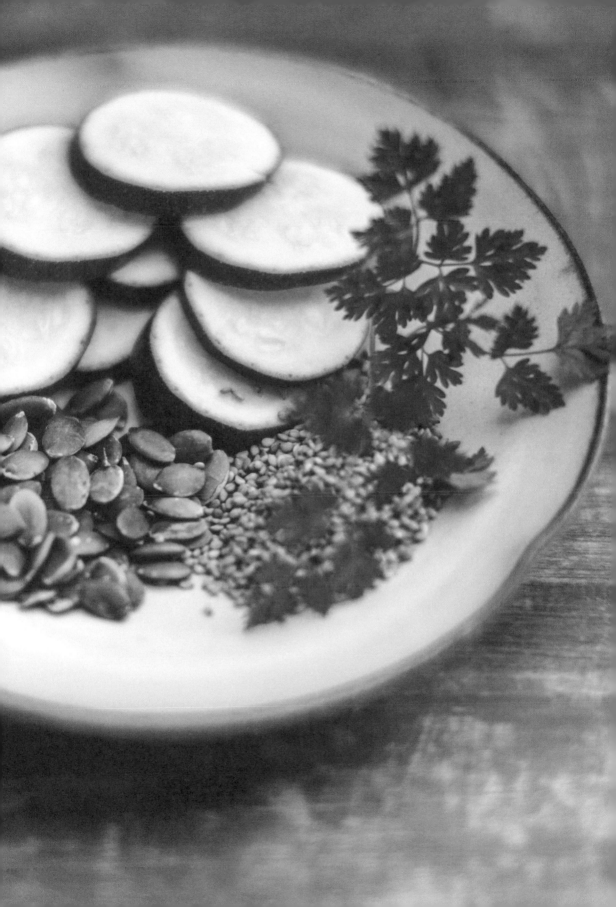

20 ALKALINE SUPERFOODS

All alkaline foods have incredible health benefits that will contribute to your overall well-being. But the alkaline superfoods listed here have been selected for their particularly high levels of beneficial alkaline ingredients.

Avocado
This creamy, highly alkaline fruit provides nearly twenty essential nutrients, including potassium, vitamin E and B vitamins, and fibre.

Pumpkin
Members of the pumpkin and squash family contain high levels of omega-3 and -6 essential fatty acids. They are also high in vitamins A and C and a number of B vitamins. Roast their seeds for a high-protein snack and use pumpkin oil in salads.

Potatoes
Rich in healthy carbohydrates, potatoes are a great source of alkalinity. Potatoes bind acids in the stomach and this alkaline effect benefits the entire body. Their nutritional profile includes vitamin C, iron, magnesium and potassium.

Amaranth
These are very small seeds, rather like poppy seeds, but tan or light brown in colour. They are notably high in the amino acid lysine, which is not true of other grains, and fibre. Just 175 grams supplies the equivalent of all the protein needed in a day. Amaranth seeds can be toasted, treated like popcorn, scattered on salads, added as a thickener in soups or used as a breakfast porridge base.

Celery

Often filled with peanut butter as the staple of children's birthday parties, celery is a valuable source of alkaline nutrition. It is particularly at home in soups and chopped over salads. It contains calcium and niacin, which means it aids digestion and lowers blood pressure.

Celeriac

Related to celery, celeriac is a root vegetable with an impressive number of vitamins, minerals and benefits. It contains B vitamins, vitamins C and K, as well as phosphorous, iron, calcium, magnesium and antioxidants. Aniseed-flavoured celeriac can be grated in salads, steamed, mashed and made into gratins.

Kale

Of all the healthy, leafy brassicas, kale is perhaps the most beneficial, boasting a long list of vitamins and minerals – especially calcium, iron, magnesium and phosphorus. Despite having a strong flavour, kale can easily be balanced with other foods to create nutritious and delicious salads, smoothies and stews.

Almonds

Not technically a true nut, the seed of the almond is what we eat. They are high in protein and calcium, as well as being a source of zinc and vitamin E. Almonds produce a calming effect and provide essential nutrients for the skin. Almond flour makes a great alternative to wheat flour for cakes and pastries.

Carrots

Carrots are packed with calcium, magnesium, potassium and beta-carotene, which metabolises into vitamin A and encourages healthy eyesight. Carrots also help to detoxify the liver and, therefore, are perfect as part of a cleansing regime.

Quinoa

Originating in the Andes, quinoa is a versatile, gluten-free seed, or 'pseudocereal'. It is exceptionally high in calcium, as well as being a rich source of fibre, magnesium and iron. It can be prepared as a meal base and then eaten hot or cold, in a similar way as one would eat rice. And considering the high protein content, nutritionally, it wins out against its more famous counterpart.

Beetroot

Beetroot is as rich in nutrients as it is in colour. A great source of folate, beetroot also contains calcium, vitamin C and potassium, among other nutrients. It has been shown to combat kidney stones, lower blood pressure and reduce the risk of cardiovascular disease.

Oils

More and more research has highlighted flaxseed (linseed) oil as one of the most beneficial oils because it provides an excellent source of omega-3 fatty acids. Cold-pressed olive, hemp, pumpkin and other nut and seed oils, have similar benefits and can bring splendid colour as well as nutritional value to your cooking.

Broccoli

This dark leafy-green vegetable of the cabbage family contains high levels of vitamin C, calcium and fibre. Broccoli serves as an antioxidant, antiviral and antibiotic liver stimulant.

Ginger

Traditionally used to combat nausea, ginger root has many other uses both in medicine and in the kitchen. It can also be made into tea or used to flavour biscuits and breads. Ginger is a source of calcium, magnesium, potassium and phosphorous, all of which improve circulation and stimulate the liver. It also acts as an antispasmodic.

Watermelon, Mango and Papaya

Watermelon is a wonderfully refreshing and hydrating fruit. Easily digested due to its high water content, it is rich in vitamins C and A, offering anti-inflammatory and antioxidant properties. Mango is a luxurious fruit, delicious on its own or in desserts and salads, and is extremely high in vitamin C and dietary fibre. The exotic papaya, with its beautifully coloured flesh, contains three times the adult daily requirement of vitamin C, providing support for the immune system and boosting skin health.

Fennel

With its fine leaves and long, slender stalks anchored by a nutritious bulb, this alkaline superfood is rich in vitamin C, fibre, potassium and manganese. It has anti-inflammatory and antioxidant properties and helps boost the immune system.

Figs

Rich in B vitamins, vitamin K, potassium, iron, magnesium and omega fatty acids, figs are a sweet way to improve your brain function, prevent cancer, build bones and protect your heart. Figs are also a source of dietary fibre. They can be enjoyed fresh (when available) or dried.

Coconut

All over the world various parts of the coconut are used for various purposes. The 'milk' can be consumed as an energising antioxidant drink, and can promote weight maintenance. The oil is a healthy alternative to other cooking oils. Coconut flesh is high in phosphorous, magnesium and potassium, and when added to various sweet and savoury dishes, can lift the flavour and add sweetness.

THE ALKALINE KITCHEN

Try to organise your kitchen to make it alkaline-friendly, so that it is easier to work in and you have the essential equipment on hand that will allow you to cook your way to a healthier lifestyle. You can, of course, cook almost anything in this book with just a knife, pan and stove, but some kits and gadgets will make life easier and cooking more fun.

If you enjoy cooking, then you will enjoy eating. The same rules apply. The kitchen should be a calm, therapeutic space. Turning it into a pleasant place to be will make you feel better, and that feeling will extend to the dishes you prepare. Food an important part of the alkaline approach and its preparation should follow the same principles of calmness and well-being.

Alkaline on a Budget
You may be surprised at how much money you will save by following an alkaline diet. A great many of the foods we recommend are reasonably inexpensive – especially vegetables, even if you are paying for premium organic produce. You can afford to pay more for herbs and buy larger quantities. Cold-pressed oils are relatively more expensive than mass-produced vegetable oils, but they are a vital component of the diet, and, again, you are only using small quantities so you can afford to build up a collection of different oils over the weeks. When buying meat or fish, try to buy the best cuts with the money you have saved from the rest of your shop.

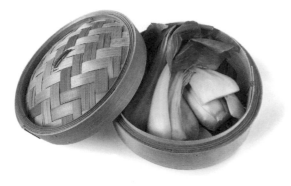

KITCHEN EQUIPMENT CHECKLIST

Steamer: Use a steamer rather than boil vegetables. Chinese-style bamboo steaming baskets are good for stacking and steaming different vegetables at the same time.

Soup pan: Large casseroles or saucepans are useful for cooking soups and stews.

Nonstick pans: With nonstick pans you do not have to use fats and oils for frying.

Grater: Graters are useful for grating zests of oranges and lemons (check that the fruits have not been waxed and wash them carefully) and vegetables for salads or soups.

Mandolin: Mandolins are useful for quickly slicing vegetables into thin leaves or uniform slices.

Coffee grinder: A coffee grinder can mill spices in the blink of an eye. You can also use an old-fashioned pestle and mortar as an alternative.

Blender: A simple, handheld stick blender is ideal for blending soups, sauces, dips and dressings.

Juicer: Juicers quickly and easily make vegetable and fruit juices.

Knives: A good knife or set of knives that are sharp are always essential items in the kitchen. A small easy-to-handle knife is vital, as well as a cleaver or larger knife for chopping root vegetables.

Strainer: Use a strainer to drain vegetables or strain liquids. You can also use a muslin cloth if you want to obtain a really clear broth.

SHOPPING

Most ingredients recommended in this book are fairly easy to find, but make sure you choose quality products, because this will make all the difference to your diet.

Vegetables and Herbs

Markets are usually the best value for buying vegetables, especially where you can buy single vegetables inexpensively. Fresh and seasonal produce is best. Organic foods are preferable because pesticides are acidic. 'Veg box' schemes offer convenience and visual affirmation of how many vegetables you should have in your kitchen each week. Herbs can be bought either as whole plants or in precut bunches.

Fruit

Buy fruit that is properly ripe. Brown spots on bananas or slight softness in fruits such as plums and peaches are obvious signs of ripeness. You can usually smell the ripeness of a melon at the base (this does not apply to watermelons).

Meat and Fish

Buy the best and the choicest leaner cuts – fillet for beef, loin for pork, cutlets and leg for lamb. Free-range chickens have more texture and flavour and are a more ethical choice than battery birds.

   With fish, fresh is best, always. Try to buy fish on the day you are going to eat it. Buying frozen fish is not necessarily a bad option because, the fish is often frozen at sea immediately after being caught and can therefore be in good condition.

Dairy and Cheese

For the alkaline cure fresh young cheeses (cow's, goat's or sheep's) made from unpasteurised milk to preserve the nutrients are preferred.

Grains and Bread

Supermarket breads are increasingly implicated in allergies and gluten intolerance. Opt for crispbread or bake your own flatbread without yeast. Grains, such as barley, quinoa and amaranth, can bring new angles to muesli and porridge and many other dishes.

ALKALINE STORE CUPBOARD BASICS

These are non-perishable foods that you will use throughout the fourteen-day alkaline cure, so make sure your store cupboard is stocked with these alkaline staples before starting.

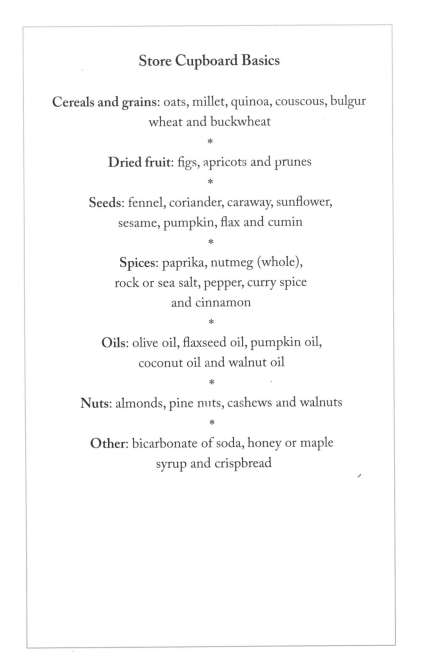

Store Cupboard Basics

Cereals and grains: oats, millet, quinoa, couscous, bulgur wheat and buckwheat

*

Dried fruit: figs, apricots and prunes

*

Seeds: fennel, coriander, caraway, sunflower, sesame, pumpkin, flax and cumin

*

Spices: paprika, nutmeg (whole), rock or sea salt, pepper, curry spice and cinnamon

*

Oils: olive oil, flaxseed oil, pumpkin oil, coconut oil and walnut oil

*

Nuts: almonds, pine nuts, cashews and walnuts

*

Other: bicarbonate of soda, honey or maple syrup and crispbread

OILS AND FATS

An alkaline kitchen should have a good range of different oils that can bring new flavours and nutrients to dishes. Oils rich in omega-3, -6 and -9 essential fatty acids are most valuable. Omega-6 is found in many different foods, including meat. We rarely need to worry about being omega-6–deficient since most of us have as much as twenty times more omega-6 other omega fatty acids. Virgin (cold-pressed) olive oil is a familiar source of omega-9, along with other nut and seed oils. Ideally, aim for a mix of one part omega-3, two parts omega-6 and one part omega-9.

Omega-3 is found mainly in flaxseed oil and oily fish. It is the omega oil that our grandmothers tried to get us to swallow by the teaspoonful.

These oils are helpful in supporting the enzymes that convert food into energy. Different oils bring different values – a good collection in an alkaline kitchen is inspiring.

The first pressing of an oil, the virgin oil, even if unfiltered, will have the most benefits. It is sometimes possible to find cold-pressed sunflower and grapeseed oils, and these have a useful role in cooking, but most budget vegetable oils have been denatured and have lost their nutritional value, and are acidic.

Maintaining Vitality

Oils are sensitive to light and should be sold in dark-coloured glass bottles or tins. Buy oils in small quantities; they are a fresh product and will lose their vitality over time. You can keep native oils for up to six months and other cold-pressed oils for up to a year.

Pumpkin Oil

Pumpkin oil is a power food that contains a rich cocktail of nutrients including vitamins A and E, zinc and selenium with an ideal blend of omega-3 and -6 essential fatty acids. In parts of eastern Europe it has earned PDO (Protected Designation of Origin) status and has been part of the diet and herbal therapies in that region for centuries. It has often been recommended for irritable bowel syndrome.

Cooking with Oil

The heat of cooking destroys many of the valuable
vitamins and omega fatty acids found in cold-pressed oils.
For that reason, add them at the end of the cooking. The
same is true of butter. Many recipes can be grilled rather
than fried. Or use a nonstick pan.

The best oil for cooking, because it has the highest
heat resistance, is coconut oil. And it is alkaline. It can be
useful when cooking Asian-style stir-fries, where its strong
flavour tends to complement the flavours
rather than overpower them.

Flaxseed Oil

In many countries in eastern Europe flaxseed (linseed) oil is used as
a dressing for potatoes and the flavour can be pronounced. In Indian
cooking it is known as *tisi*. It is rich in omega-3 essential fatty acids.
Cultivation goes back to the Neolithic era, when flax was widely used
to make linen.

Hempseed Oil

Hemp or hempseed oil has a grassy, nutty taste that increases the
darker it is. Not to be confused with the intoxicating hash oil, which is
made from the flowers and leaves of the plant, the oil from the seeds is
of high nutritional value because of its 3:1 ratio of omega-6 to omega-3
essential fatty acids – an ideal blend. It also contains vitamin D and
high levels of vitamin E.

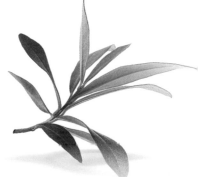

HOW TO COOK

In this programme we recommend short cooking times, because we have learned that overheating food can destroy valuable proteins, enzymes and nutrients. Herbs, in fact, should never be cooked but only incorporated at the very end of the cooking process. Our restaurant at the clinic enjoys a deserved gastronomic reputation and that is because we see no contradiction between food that tastes good and food that is good for us.

Cooking should be therapeutic and enjoyable, a part of the rhythm of life. It is a good way to create breaks in the day and the evening when you have time to leave other things behind. Just as with eating, you need to set aside time to prepare the ingredients properly. Cooking should not be rushed nor be stressful. Preparing a good soup can be a pleasurable process; enjoy handling the raw vegetables and transforming them into something to look forward to.

Cook vegetables for as short a time as possible. A useful tip is to cut vegetables into small pieces or even grate them so that they cook faster.

Stock is often a hurdle for cooks, but in the alkaline kitchen it is easy – just reserve the water in which you have cooked your vegetables and then you will always have a continual supply of fresh stock for poaching or for making soups, which will add extra nutritional goodness. Cooking can, and should be, a cyclical process.

Breaking the Frying Habit

Poaching or simmering is healthy and can often replace frying, which is perhaps more of a habit than a necessity. Deep-fat frying is, by definition, an acidifying process. From an alkaline perspective, most recipes that begin with frying vegetables are to be avoided. Grilling is a cleaner option for meat. Steaming vegetables is better than boiling them. Baking, which essentially is just dry poaching, is equally acceptable for the alkaline cure.

Butter should not be exposed to too much heat when cooking; therefore, a knob on boiled potatoes after cooking is fine, especially along with a few chopped chives or parsley.

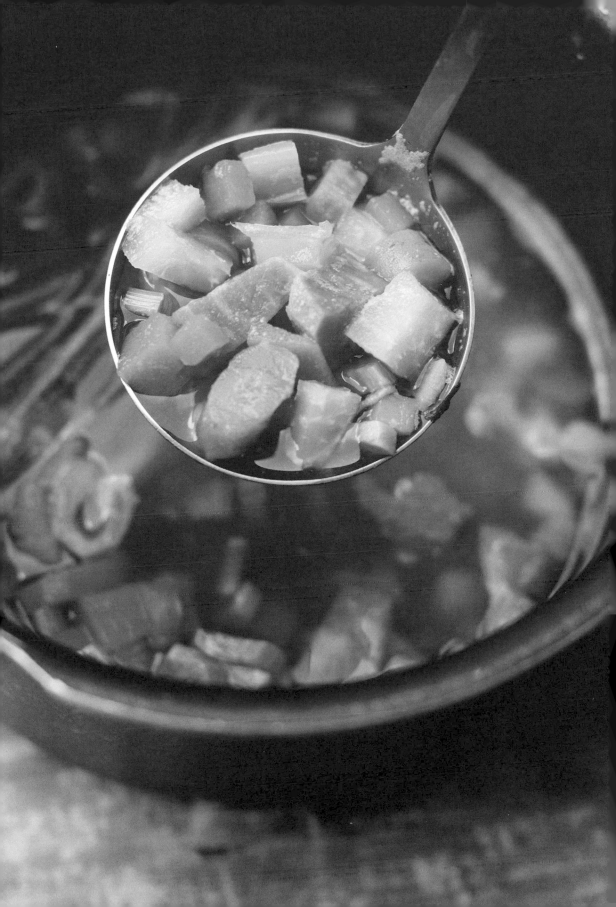

Heaping on the Herbs

Herbs should be used as abundantly as you can, either while cooking or sprinkled over a dish before serving. Be extravagant. These are permitted luxuries, so try to enjoy them.

Asian influences offer us many sensible ideas in the kitchen. In Thai cuisine, the holy trinity of seasoning is garlic, ginger and chilli – all alkalising influences. In Asian cuisine dishes are garnished not with one or two leaves but handfuls of coriander and basil.

When cooking with herbs, there are a few things to keep in mind: basil does not like heat at all, so only add it to dishes at the last minute; rosemary and thyme have strong flavours and are most suited for broths and teas; sage and marjoram are great complementary herbs for poultry and other meats; chervil adds a delicate flair to dishes.

Keep fresh herbs in jars or cups with the stems in water, in the same way as a bouquet of flowers. Change the water regularly. Dried herbs and seeds should be stored in dark, cool places.

Spicing Up Your Life

Spices can be toasted in a frying pan or dried in the oven quickly and mixed with rock salt to dramatically change the nature of a dish. The typical ingredients of store-bought curry powder are mostly alkaline – coriander seed, cayenne pepper, cumin, garlic, ginger – although you may prefer to make up your own and avoid any preservatives bottled mixes may contain. A coffee grinder doubles up as a spice mill, and if you make too much you can always store it and use it as and when needed.

Rock and sea salts provide minerals to the diet. Most types of salt taste very different. Much of the sodium impact will depend on the size of the grain or flake, which can also offer textures. A good collection of different salts, such as homemade blends of salt and herbs, are fine additions to your kitchen staples.

Whole Foods Versus Purées

Puréed soups and dips offer the fastest, most efficient way of delivering nutritional benefits. Vegetables prepared in this way are easier to digest than whole vegetables, and vegetable purées can be vehicles for different flavourings, especially herbs, spices and even omega-rich oils. And for meals later in the day when the body might not have enough time to break down solids, they can play a useful role.

But for most of us, the fibre in foods is also an important aspect of eating and helping teach the body how to digest. From this point of view, whole vegetables are better. But it is also a question of balance. For example, take an orange. It may take upwards of three or four oranges to make a glass of orange juice. That represents a major nutritional impact compared to eating a few slices of orange. However, the body's digestive system is more comfortable with the orange slices as opposed to the glass of pulped juice with a vitamin content that is sixteen times greater. You may feel as if you're getting a whole lot of vitamins, but your body may not agree or be able to benefit from it.

Preserving

Fresh foods are always preferable. The issues with preserving foods from a nutritional point of view are obvious and go further than just concerns about histamine. In extending storage life, fruits, vegetables and other high-value sources of nutrition inevitably degrade.

Agents used for preserving food – most commonly salt, sugar, vinegar and other additives – are acidic. With very few exceptions, any foods sold in bags, cans, sleeves or other kinds of packaging are very likely to be more acid. Even a microwave dinner that contains ingredients that seem to have an alkaline leaning, when filled with preservatives and packaged, themselves become acidic.

Better to use fresh ingredients and cook a meal yourself. Frozen vegetables without additives, especially chestnuts, corn and peas, may remain alkaline, but mixes of ingredients for meals are unlikely to sustain their much-needed alkalinity.

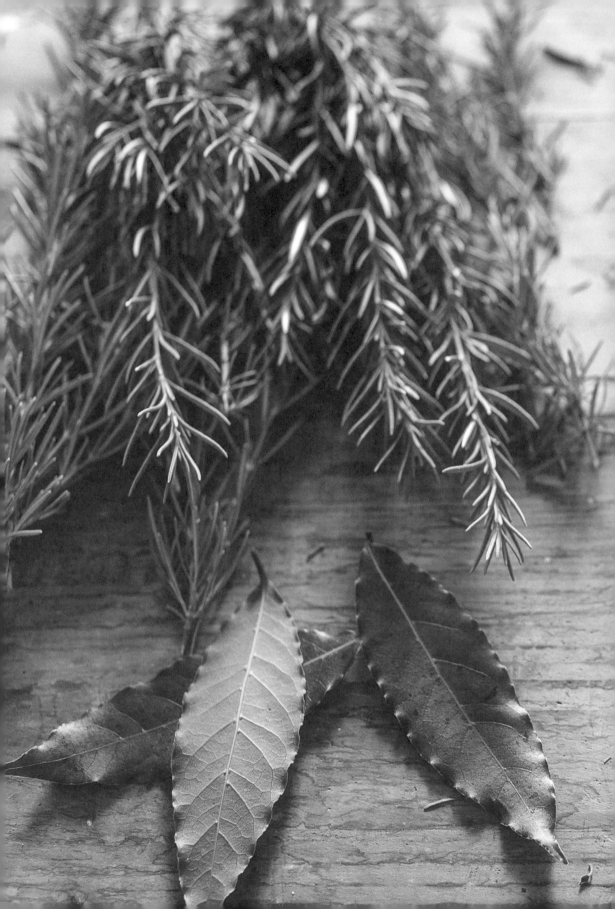

5

The Fourteen-Day Alkaline Cure

Getting Started
Week One Shopping List
Days One to Seven
Building on Your Cure
Week Two Shopping List
Days Eight to Fourteen
After the Cure

GETTING STARTED

The best time to start your alkaline cure is on a weekend or a day when you are not going to be distracted so you can give yourself enough time to get organised. Keep things simple and straightforward and do what is manageable for your schedule. If you prepare your breakfast the night before, you will have all the elements easily to hand without having to think about it in the morning. Also, if you make up your vegetable tea or soup the night before, it will have time to infuse.

Depending on how acidic your body is, you are likely to feel some side effects as you go: headaches, fatigue, anxiety, mood changes or cravings. These are good signs, indicating that your body is getting rid of toxins. Live with them. They will pass quickly enough. Remember that many of our health problems have built up over several years, and real change may take time. The next fourteen days is a start.

THE WEEK BEFORE YOU START

You might reward yourself with a couple of days off from work to get yourself up and running. Pencil a date in your calendar and give yourself a few days to get used to the idea. It is also a good idea to adopt a few new changes before starting the programme:

* Cut down on coffee, alcohol and carbonated drinks.

* If you're interested in monitoring your pH during the cure, purchase pH testing litmus strips.

* Don't buy any fast food, junk food and packaged food. Clean out your refrigerator and store cupboard to remove temptation and replace acid foods with suitable snacks.

* Cut out sugar, especially refined sugar, and begin to load your body up with nutrients. Your body will need plenty of extra nutrients during the cure and eating healthier foods before you begin will make the transition less extreme.

* Start drinking water and get into the habit of drinking two litres or more a day.

* Make a shopping list for the first few days so you have everything to hand at home. Do not be tempted to economise on your shopping – the best, freshest produce will create the tastiest, healthiest meals. Your food portions over the next two weeks will be fairly controlled, so you should be able to afford to be a little extravagant with the quality of your ingredients.

* One tip that can help you to start eating less is to use smaller plates. Serve your meals on side plates or in bowls rather than on full-size dinner plates.

* Start establishing a relaxing new evening routine. For instance, take a walk after dinner and give yourself some personal time to read a book. Take a warm bath two hours before you go to bed.

THE DAY BEFORE YOU START

The day before you start the plan, go shopping and get everything ready in the kitchen. Make an alkaline minestrone (page 142) so you know you have a good, dependable standby waiting for you to enjoy. All of the recipes in the day planner can be found in the section 6, listed by category and in order of appearance in the programme. For ease of reference, there is a recipe finder at the back of the book. It's not crucial to get all the ingredients to follow the recipes precisely; just buy produce according to the seasons and use your judgement to substitute equivalent alkaline vegetables, spices and herbs.

If you are or want to be a vegetarian, substitute the meat-based recipes in the day planner with any of the menu options that are marked with a ⓥ in the recipe section.

Since exercise is such an important part of the alkaline cure, the evening before you begin, take a stroll outside. We have provided you with new exercises to try every day that alternate between cardio, stretching, breathing and core-strengthening exercises. We have also given beauty and environment tips to help you create an alkaline lifestyle. The 'In the Kitchen' section of the day planner has suggestions for dishes you can make in the evening for the following day.

DAILY ACTIVITIES

A daily routine is good. While taking the alkaline
cure, try to do the following every day:

* **Dry brush your skin:** Before your daily bath or shower,
  take a loofah or natural bristle brush and gently dry brush
  your skin. This will eliminate dead skin cells, unblock pores,
  kickstart the lymph system and increase blood circulation.

* **Rinse your mouth with flaxseed oil:** An oil mouthwash is
  an effective way of cleaning your palate. Use flaxseed oil or
  another kind of nut or seed oil for a few minutes to rinse
  away any toxins in the gums and to protect against gum
  disease. Not all toxins will dissolve in water so rinse your
  mouth with oil regularly.

* **Do thirty minutes of exercise:** Try to get at least thirty
  minutes of exercise per day. This may seem like a daunting
  task, but even something as simple as taking the stairs
  rather than the lift contributes to your thirty minutes.
  Exercise comes in many different forms: a brisk walk,
  a bike ride, a game of tennis, a yoga class, a swim. It
  shouldn't be difficult to find something that works for
  you and your lifestyle.

* **Keep hydrated:** By drinking water, vegetable tea or herbal
  tea throughout the day, you can keep your body properly
  hydrated. Aim to drink at least two litres a day. Keep
  vegetable tea to hand so you have something refreshing
  and nutritious to enjoy at any time of day.

Week One

The aim in week one is to cleanse the system of toxins with a minimum of stress on the system. The menu is designed to bring the digestive system back into harmony, flushing out the acids and focusing on simple, cleansing foods. The planner also includes daily exercises and beauty and environment tips for every other day.

WEEK ONE SHOPPING LIST

The shopping list below is to help you organise your first week
of meals based on the menus we've listed in the day planner for days
one to seven. The following list is for one person. If you are feeding
more, increase the quantities proportionally.

Fresh Basics
*These are fresh foods you
will use through the week, so
buy as needed*

Fresh herbs: parsley, rosemary,
sage, thyme, basil, mint, lovage,
coriander, dill, nettle, yarrow,
lemon balm, lemon verbena,
chamomile and bay leaves

*

Vegetables, fruits and roots:
ginger root, potatoes, fennel,
juniper berries, turnips, celery,
broccoli, green onions, courgettes,
fresh horseradish, lemons, carrots
and parsnips

*

Milk products: milk (or soy
milk or almond milk), curd,
plain yogurt, goat's or
sheep's cheese and butter

*

Other: eggs, spelt bread and
crispbread

Days One and Two

1 chicken breast (85 g)

*

4 new potatoes

*

Green beans

*

Salad leaves

*

Parmesan (grated)

*

1 aubergine

*

Pitted black olives

Days Three and Four

1 tuna fillet (85 g)

*

1 beef fillet (85 g)

*

1 avocado

*

1 lime

*

1 sweet potato

*

1 apple

*

1 baking potato

*

Currants

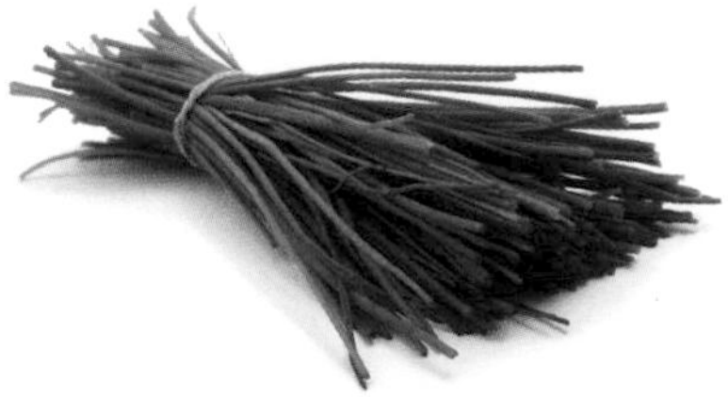

Days Five, Six and Seven

1 salmon fillet (85 g)

*

1 avocado

*

1 apple

*

1 beetroot

*

1 aubergine

*

1 can of broad beans

*

Pitted black olives

*

Spinach

*

1 tomato

*

Dill

*

Currants

*

Chives

DAY ONE
Sunday

Take it slowly. One step at a time. You do not need to change the world before six o'clock. Give yourself a chance to welcome new ideas and get into a new mood, a new rhythm. Take your time. Calm is good. Speed is stressful. Put the brakes on...

WAKE UP
Hot water with lemon or
rosemary tea

BREAKFAST
Mediterranean vegetable spread
on spelt toast or crispbread

LUNCH
Grilled chicken with baby
potatoes, broccoli and carrots

DINNER
Alkaline minestrone

BEDTIME
Lemon balm tea

Recipes can be found in section 6

Cardio Exercise

Regular cardio exercise is an important part of the programme. Today, go for a brisk walk. Your pace should be fast enough that you feel your heart beating and your respiratory rate increasing. Try to walk at this pace for half an hour.

Beauty – Avocado Hair Mask

Peel and mash a ripe avocado in a bowl. Mix in a tablespoon of honey. Apply the mix to your hair and cover your head with a shower cap. Leave the hair mask on for twenty minutes and then rinse. This mask will leave your hair looking and feeling lustrous.

In the Kitchen

Soak dried figs in hot herbal tea for tomorrow's breakfast.
Liquidise your alkaline minestrone so it is a purée for tomorrow's lunch.
Make almond pesto.
Prepare Mayr vegetable tea.

'Awareness is the conscious focusing on the moment. Perception and acceptance make us view the world as if it's in slow motion. Our environment and our own reactions become clearer.'

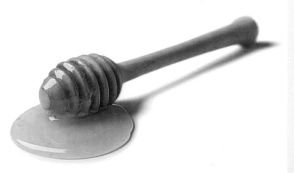

DAY TWO
Monday

Chewing is crucial to getting the most out of your food. It is a fundamental part of the alkaline cure. Chewing effectively makes up for the smaller quantity of food. The better you chew, the better you will digest and extract the maximum amount of nutrition from your food. Try to chew each mouthful thirty times.

WAKE UP
Hot water with lemon or
ginger tea

BREAKFAST
Fresh yogurt with flaxseed
Figs poached in herbal tea

LUNCH
Salad of green beans, potatoes
and mixed leaves in olive oil

DINNER
Puréed alkaline minestrone
Almond pesto

BEDTIME
Lemon balm tea

Recipes can be found in section 6

Stretching – Stomach Exercise

This stretch is good for your core abdominal muscles because it changes the pivotal point in the stomach. It also puts a different kind of pressure on the gut and works like an internal massage.

Lying down on your back, bring your knees up against your chest, then rotate your body – knees to the left, head to the right. Alternate.

Environment
Listen to calming music that you enjoy – perhaps something choral or classical. Maybe find a new piece to listen to in the evenings. Discover new composers and genres to go with your diet.

In the Kitchen
Make celery soup for tomorrow's dinner.
Soak dried figs in hot herbal tea for tomorrow's breakfast.

'Even the most alkaline recipes will turn acid in your stomach if you do not chew. Food should be savoured and enjoyed slowly.'

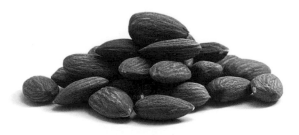

DAY THREE
Tuesday

The old saying was you should breakfast like a king, lunch like a prince and dine like a pauper. You can be a little lavish in the morning because your body has all day to digest, but be careful not to eat too much or you will make yourself feel hungrier later. The more you give your stomach, the more it wants. Give it less.

WAKE UP
Hot water with lemon or
thyme tea

BREAKFAST
Power muesli
Figs poached in herbal tea

LUNCH
Seared tuna, avocado, ginger,
coriander and lime

DINNER
Celery soup

BEDTIME
Yarrow tea

Recipes can be found in section 6

Relaxation – Breathing Exercise

This is a gentle breathing exercise that will calm both your mind and your spirit.

Sit in a comfortable, upright position and bring one hand close to your mouth, with the thumb and index fingers together, as if holding the end of a feather. Purse your lips and inhale slowly through your mouth. Then blow out gently, making a soft 'hoo' sound, as if blowing an imaginary feather. Your fingertips should feel a cool breeze.

Repeat until you feel very calm and cool.

Beauty – Alkaline Bath

Add 130 g bicarbonate of soda to your bath with. Use a pH indicator to check the water for a pH of 8.5. Soak for thirty to sixty minutes. As your skin wrinkles it will become soft and allow the acids to get out. This treatment is often used to treat arthritis and rheumatic diseases.

In the Kitchen

Assemble your omega mix for tomorrow's breakfast.
Prepare Mayr vegetable tea.

'If you feel like sitting down on the sofa after eating, that is a bad sign, a sign that you are eating the wrong things. After a meal, you should feel light, alert, full of energy.'

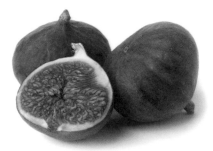

DAY FOUR
Wednesday

Change is good, for both the mind and the body. Exercise to move parts of the body you have forgotten about, especially the core. This is the new you.

WAKE UP
Hot water with lemon or
sage tea

BREAKFAST
Fresh yogurt with honey and
omega mix

LUNCH
Fillet of beef with braised celery and
mashed sweet potato

DINNER
Baked potato with butter and chives

BEDTIME
Yarrow tea

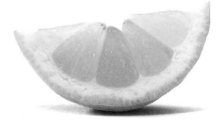

Recipes can be found in section 6

Strengthening – Core Exercise

This exercise will strengthen your core muscles and improve your breathing by opening your chest.

Sit on the floor with your knees bent to the left side of your body and tuck your feet close to your right hip. Place your right foot into the arch of your left foot. Lengthen your spine, sit up tall and turn your torso to the left. Reach across your body with your right arm and place it on your left knee. Stretch your left arm behind you and place it on the floor. Untwist into the centre position.

Repeat three times before changing sides.

Environment

Buy some colourful flowers and place them around your home where you can appreciate them: in the bathroom, your bedroom and the kitchen.

In the Kitchen

Make alkaline minestrone for tomorrow's dinner.

Prepare Mediterranean vegetable spread for tomorrow's breakfast.

Soak dried figs in hot herbal tea for tomorrow's breakfast.

'If you move, you breathe off the acids building up in your body. The lungs ventilate; the acids offload. Motion is key. Any kind of motion is positive.'

DAY FIVE
Thursday

Eating is about quality not quantity. The right foods at the right time. Take your time when eating: put your knife and fork down between mouthfuls, appreciate what you are doing. Allow yourself a generous amount of time to eat, too — at least thirty minutes eating time, not including preparation.

WAKE UP
Hot water with lemon or
peppermint tea

BREAKFAST
Figs poached in herbal tea
Mediterranean vegetable spread
on spelt toast or crispbread

LUNCH
Quinoa salad with avocado, tomato,
parsley and pine nuts
Olive oil dressing

DINNER
Alkaline minestrone

BEDTIME
Chamomile tea

Recipes can be found in section 6

Cardio Exercise

If you have a pool or a swimming complex nearby, go for a half-hour swim. Swimming is a low-impact cardio activity that works many muscle groups at once, stretching and strengthening your muscles. In the water, try different strokes and kicks. Swimming is not only good for your heart and muscles, it can also relieve sore joints.

Beauty – Sea Salt Scrub

Mix Dead Sea salt and almond oil together and gently exfoliate your body. Rinse with warm water and pat dry. A salt scrub removes dead skin cells and bacteria, improves circulation and encourages cell regeneration.

In the Kitchen

Prepare sheep's cheese and horseradish spread for tomorrow's dinner.
Make herb soup for tomorrow's dinner.
Prepare Mayr vegetable tea.

'Eat enough. Sufficiently. You can train your body to live on less. It does not need more. That is life prolonging in itself.'

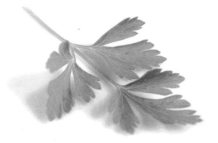

DAY SIX
Friday

Herbs come from the earth and so they bring with them their own minerality. Each herb has its own season and time of the year and makes its own contribution to your nutrition. Use them generously; they are valuable.

WAKE UP
Hot water with lemon or
nettle tea

BREAKFAST
Herb omelette

LUNCH
Poached salmon,
Carrot and spinach mash
and hemp sauce

DINNER
Herb soup
Sheep's cheese and horseradish spread
on spelt toast or crispbread

BEDTIME
Chamomile tea

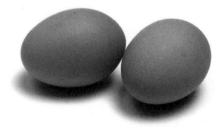

Recipes can be found in section 6

Stretching – Yoga Exercise

This yoga pose, called the Tree Pose, will help improve your balance, memory and concentration by engaging both your body and mind.

Stand in an upright position – feet firmly planted to the floor, knees locked, back straight and tall. Balance on one leg. Draw the opposite foot to the thigh or calf of the standing leg, never against the knee. Concentrate, and raise your hands above your head. Remember to breathe; it will only interfere with your balance if you don't. Keep your hips even by lowering the position of your foot on your inner thigh.

Hold for five deep breaths, then slowly come out of the posture. Change sides.

Environment

Switch off the television and your computer, and put your mobile phone aside. Try to enjoy a relaxing evening without the buzz of the outside world.

In the Kitchen

Make spinach and nutmeg soup for tomorrow's dinner.

'Bitterness is good. It is a sign of a natural, pure product – roots are bitter, and bitter plants like artichoke are helpful for the liver. So are radicchio and chicory. Herbs tend to be bitter. Dandelion is good, too, as are nettles in spring. Our liking for sweet things stems from our mother's milk, which was sweet. But as we get older, we need other things.'

DAY SEVEN
Saturday

By now you should be feeling the benefits of changing your diet and enjoying lots of new foods and flavours – your body should also be feeling healthier and fitter. You have worked hard all week and have earned a relaxing day.

WAKE UP
Hot water with lemon or
lemon verbena tea

BREAKFAST
Power muesli

LUNCH
Roasted beetroot, broad beans
and chives with walnut oil

DINNER
Spinach and nutmeg soup

BEDTIME
Fennel tea

Recipes can be found in section 6

Exercise
It's your seventh day and you've done well. This evening, take a relaxing stroll after dinner.

Treat
Take a steam at a sauna.

Beauty – Alkaline Footbath
Fill a small tub with warm water mixed with bicarbonate of soda. Bicarbonate of soda has many benefits, including skin smoothing and has an antifungal action.

In the Kitchen
Make leek and potato soup for tomorrow's dinner.
Prepare Mayr vegetable tea.
Soak millet and buckwheat flakes for tomorrow's breakfast.

'You are your best doctor. I can only guide you. You know yourself better than I do. You know your body. You just have to be aware of bad influences. The more you can program yourself and your responses with alkaline messages, the easier it will become to identify and listen to what your body is saying. Listen to your body. Have a talk with it.'

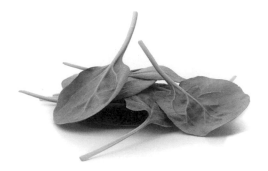

BUILDING ON YOUR CURE

After a week of gentle cleansing, your body should be responding and you may notice that what you are eating tastes better. In the past seven days, depending on your previous lifestyle, you may have experienced severe headaches, anxiety, mood changes and cravings. At the clinic we usually say that it takes at least ten days for all of the benefits to start to kick in, but you should already begin to notice some positive changes occurring after this first week. Generally, you should be feeling more energized, your skin should be looking clearer, and you should be feeling more regular and less constipated and bloated.

Balancing Week

In your second week you will be introduced to some more ideas that will make cooking and eating more enjoyable and give you a head start on the alkaline way of life. While in the first week was on nursing your system back to health, this week the aim is to stimulate your body and mind and create a new kind of balance.

Little things matter. A scattering of sesame or sunflower seeds can spice up a breakfast; a drizzle of pumpkin oil or flaxseed oil can bring new elements to plain curd or yogurt. This week, make good use of your alkaline store cupboard and, with it, build up new levels of flavour and nutrition at every meal.

As you continue with the plan, remember to keep yourself hydrated – two litres or more of water a day will help to wash out the toxins in your system and keep your body working properly.

Week Two

This week you can open up and explore some new and different foods to add to the cleansing foods you ate last week. The recipes are still easy to follow but use a wider spectrum of ingredients for fuller, more creative meals. The more different alkaline foods we eat, the more our bodies can take advantage of the nutritional benefits they offer.

WEEK TWO SHOPPING LIST

The shopping list below is to help you organise your second week of meals based on the menus listed in the day planner for days eight to fourteen. The following list is for one person. If you are feeding more, increase the quantities proportionally.

Fresh Basics

These are fresh foods you will use throughout the week, so buy as needed

Fresh herbs: parsley, rosemary, sage, thyme, basil, mint, lovage, coriander, dill, nettle, yarrow, lemon balm, lemon verbena, chamomile and bay

*

Vegetables, fruits and roots: ginger root, potatoes, fennel, juniper berries, turnips, celery, broccoli, green onions, courgettes, fresh horseradish, lemons, carrots and parsnips

*

Milk products: milk (or soy milk or almond milk), curd, plain yogurt, goat's or sheep's cheese and butter

*

Other: eggs, spelt bread and crispbread

Days Eight and Nine

Smoked mackerel (85 g)

*

1 grapefruit

*

1 artichoke

*

2 shiitake mushrooms

*

10 mangetout pods

*

5 leeks

*

1 pak choi

*

Lemongrass

*

Green beans

*

Coconut milk

*

Rice noodles or tofu

*

Cream or crème fraîche

*

Chives

*

Mustard

Days Ten,
Eleven and Twelve

Minced beef
(85 g; buy on Day 11)
*
1 orange
*
1 grapefruit
*
Strawberries
*
1 avocado
*
1 red pepper
*
1 aubergine
*
1 sweet potato
*
1 garlic bulb
*
Pitted black olives
*
1 kohlrabi
*
1 celeriac
*
1 cucumber
*
Cream
*
3 chestnuts

Days Thirteen and Fourteen

1 lamb chop (85 g)
*
1 lime
*
2 avocados
*
2 fresh figs
*
1 small melon of choice
*
Berries of choice
*
1 cucumber
*
1 beetroot

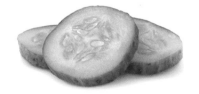

DAY EIGHT
Sunday

Today is a spice day. Historically, spices were used as medicine to perk up the system. Many spices still form the basis of our modern medicine and they bring benefits to your diet that may be neglected in your daily meals. In their natural form, they have a valuable role to play.

WAKE UP
Hot water with lemon or
rosemary tea

BREAKFAST
Millet and buckwheat porridge
with cinnamon and ginger

LUNCH
Asian-style stir-fry

DINNER
Leek and potato soup

BEDTIME
Fennel tea

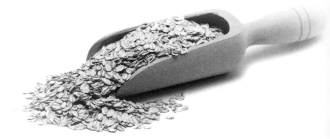

Recipes can be
found in section 6

Relaxation – Breathing Exercise

Create your own breathing sequence using all three of these upper-body breathing exercises: for abdomen, for chest and for shoulders. Try to do it outside or in front of an open window.

Sitting down with your back straight, put your fingers on your stomach. Breathe in hard with your belly so you can feel the effect on your diaphragm – your fingers should move apart. Repeat ten times, taking long and slow breaths.

Sitting down with your back straight, bring your fingers up to your chest. Breathe in deeply, feel the strength of your lungs. Exhale slowly. Repeat ten times.

Place your hands on your collarbones and breathe in, concentrating on the whole of the upper body. Breathe out and relax. Take twenty of these breaths.

Environment

Before you go to bed, turn off the alarm clock and let your body decide how much sleep you really need. Aim to wake up naturally at dawn.

In the Kitchen

Prepare curd and paprika spread for tomorrow's breakfast.

'The only supplement I might recommend that you cannot always find in your diet is zinc. The importance of zinc is that it forces the body to produce bicarbonate naturally. However, it is mostly found in oysters and red meats. You can be low on zinc without noticing, although it is often seen in poor hair and brittle nails.'

DAY NINE
Monday

The oils that you have been using throughout the week provide essential fatty acids in your diet. They are the switches that turn what we eat into nutrition. Blend and vary the oils you use. Flaxseed oil is the most valuable because it is high in omega-3 fatty acids and makes a great base oil for many recipes. But if you don't like the flavour, other nut oils, olive oils and organic seed oils can be used as they are also immensely important.

WAKE UP
Hot water with lemon or
ginger tea

BREAKFAST
Grapefruit Curd and paprika spread
on spelt toast or crispbread

LUNCH
Artichoke hearts with flaxseed
and herb vinaigrette

DINNER
Smoked mackerel and
vegetables with parsley oil

BEDTIME
Lemon balm tea

Recipes can be found in section 6

Strengthening – Core Exercise

This exercise will help improve your coordination, which plays a major role in core strengthening.

Kneel on your hands and knees, holding weights in both hands. Form a straight line from your shoulders to your hands and from your hips to your knees. Stretch one leg out straight behind your torso on the floor while stretching your opposite arm on the floor in front of you. Lift your extended arm and leg up to shoulder and hip level. Keep your palm down. Lower your arm and leg to the floor.

Lift and lower five times and then change sides.

Beauty – Warm Liver Compress

Apply a warm compress to your liver before you go to bed. Wrap a dampened tea towel around a hot-water bottle filled with warm water. Lie back and place it underneath your ribs and to the right. Leave for fifteen minutes or even all night.

In the Kitchen

Make carrot and ginger soup for tomorrow's dinner.
Prepare Mediterranean vegetable spread for tomorrow's dinner.
Prepare Mayr vegetable tea.

*'Sweating is good. Train your body to sweat.
You are getting rid of the acids.'*

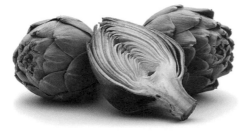

DAY TEN
Tuesday

Most of us have developed a habit of eating too much. Cut your portion sizes down. At restaurants, do not be tempted to eat everything on your plate. At home, use small plates rather than big ones. Vary your diet with different foods to keep meal times interesting. Eat slowly so that you take the same amount of time for dinner but eat less. Put your cutlery down between mouthfuls.

WAKE UP
Hot water with lemon or
thyme tea

BREAKFAST
Fresh yogurt with honey and
omega mix

LUNCH
Baked pepper stuffed with bulgur wheat
and nuts

DINNER
Carrot and ginger soup
Mediterranean vegetable spread
on spelt toast or crispbread

BEDTIME
Lemon balm tea

Recipes can be found in section 6

Cardio Exercise

Today, go for a jog or use a cross-trainer in the gym for at least half an hour. Try to vary your pace while jogging: every five minutes, increase your pace by thirty per cent for a minute and then reduce it.

Environment

Buy some houseplants. They will improve the oxygen levels in your home and give a calming feel to your décor.

In the Kitchen

Soak dried apricots in hot herbal tea for tomorrow's breakfast.
Prepare herb spread for tomorrow's dinner.

'If you cannot sleep, treat it as an advantage. You have more time in the day. Relax and enjoy the sweet and tranquil rhythm of your thoughts. Watch them go by without interfering. Go with the flow. You do not need to sleep to be relaxed and rested.'

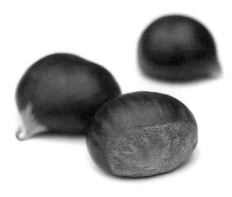

DAY ELEVEN
Wednesday

Keep up your routines – exercising, preparing meals, dry skin brushing, bathing, sleeping. Routine is immensely powerful. The body prepares itself better if your life is regular. Hormones have a twenty-four-hour cycle and are easily disturbed. In order to reset their balance, you need to have a regular routine.

WAKE UP
Hot water with lemon or
sage tea

BREAKFAST
Goat's cheese on spelt toast or crispbread
Apricots poached in herbal tea

LUNCH
Spicy meatballs with tzatziki
Strawberries

DINNER
Warm salad of kohlrabi,
broccoli and celeriac in herb oil
Herb spread on spelt toast or crispbread

BEDTIME
Yarrow tea

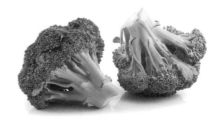

Recipes can be found in section 6

Relaxation – Breathing Exercise

Sit in a comfortable upright position. Close your eyes and breathe naturally. Rest your right hand on your right knee, keeping your hand relaxed and open.

Raise your left hand and place your thumb gently against your left nostril. Breathe in slowly, taking a full breath through your right nostril. Gently close your right nostril with the fourth finger of your left hand. Hold for a second, then slowly release the fourth finger and breathe out through your right nostril until your lungs are empty.

Repeat five times and then change sides, inhaling and exhaling through your left nostril. Repeat five times.

Beauty – Alkaline Face Mask

You can make an easy alkaline face mask with curd or quark and honey. Honey is an antimicrobial and an antioxidant while curd soothes. Combine a teaspoon of each, apply and leave for ten minutes before rinsing.

In the Kitchen

Make fennel and dill soup for tomorrow's dinner.
Prepare herb spread (if more is needed).
Prepare Mayr vegetable tea.

'Breathing helps to make us aware of our bodies. It helps us to focus on the core, the abdomen, the torso and not always think of our bodies as arms and legs. Even in the office, take five minutes, open a window, put your hands on your knees, and breathe in at different tempos – fast like laughing, slow and deep to create rhythm. Follow your heartbeat, remember who you are.'

DAY TWELVE
Thursday

As you near the end of your fourteen-day plan, your body should be enjoying its natural rhythms and processes. You should be starting to feel less stressed, more energised and more positive. You will find that eating alkaline is starting to become second nature, rather than a regime you have to consciously adhere to. You will start to associate healthy food with feeling good and stop craving the unhealthy foods you may have craved before.

WAKE UP
Hot water with lemon or
peppermint tea

BREAKFAST
Grapefruit
Millet and buckwheat porridge
with cinnamon and ginger

LUNCH
Quinoa risotto

DINNER
Fennel and dill soup
Herb spread on spelt toast or crispbread

BEDTIME
Yarrow tea

Recipes can be found in section 6

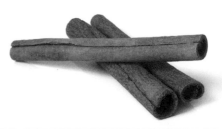

Strengthening — Core Exercise

This exercise, called spine curls, requires you to peel your spine off the floor vertebra by vertebra. Doing this slowly will help further strengthen your core muscles.

Lie flat on your back with your knees bent and your feet on the floor hip-width apart. Breathe in. As you breathe out, tilt your pelvis so that your lower back sinks into the mat and your pubic bone lifts towards the ceiling. Breathe in. Breathe out as you lower yourself back down.

Repeat, lifting a little more of your spine off the floor each time until you have lifted your whole abdomen up to your shoulder blades. Hold and breathe in. As you breathe out, gently reverse the movement.

Environment

You have cleansed your system, now clean out your home. Get rid of things you don't need and establish an orderly living environment.

In the Kitchen

Prepare sheep's cheese and horseradish spread for tomorrow's breakfast.

'Turn off all the electronics in your bedroom. The best light for us is still candlelight. Our ancestors gathered around an open fire to meet and to talk and that is still the most positive kind of light we are attuned to.'

DAY THIRTEEN
Friday

Listen to your body's rhythms and learn to adapt to a better lifestyle. Your body will naturally tell you what it needs, but you have to recognise the good signals and not slip back into bad habits. For instance, if your body feels tired and you're not at work or doing something important, lie down and have a nap. Be a friend to yourself and your body.

WAKE UP
Hot water with lemon or
nettle tea

BREAKFAST
Melon
Sheep's cheese and horseradish spread
on spelt toast or crispbread

LUNCH
Gratin of potatoes, onion and nutmeg

DINNER
Roasted beet with walnut oil and caraway seeds
Braised fennel with courgettes

BEDTIME
Chamomile tea

Recipes can be found in section 6

Cardio Exercise

Today, go for a bike ride either on a bike outside or on a stationary bike. Aim to go for half an hour and try to challenge yourself with different inclines and gears. Cycling will tone and strengthen your legs, thighs and glutes. It is a lower impact activity than running and it can also relieve back pain and muscle strain in your feet and knees.

Beauty – Milk and
Honey Bath
Add two litres of milk and 350 grams of honey to a warm bath. Soak for at least fifteen minutes. Afterwards, your skin will look radiant and feel like silk.

In the Kitchen
Prepare Mayr vegetable tea.
Make alkaline minestrone for
   tomorrow's dinner.
Prepare avocado spread for
   tomorrow's breakfast.

'Potassium is essential in pushing out the acids through the body. As soon as you are alkaline, the vegetables you eat facilitate the benefits to the body.'

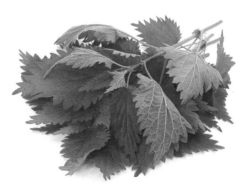

DAY FOURTEEN
Saturday

Well done! You should be feeling energised and revitalised – a new you. Enjoy your new vitality and reflect on all the changes you have made in the past two weeks. Don't beat yourself up if there are still things you wish to change. Remember, you are you, and now you're off to a wonderful new start. Remember to keep going and you will surprise yourself with how good you can feel.

WAKE UP
Hot water with lemon or
lemon verbena tea

BREAKFAST
Fresh berries and melon
Avocado spread on spelt toast or crispbread

LUNCH
Grilled lamb chop with fennel,
cucumber, grapefruit and fig salad

DINNER
Alkaline minestrone

BEDTIME
Chamomile tea

Recipes can be found in section 6

Exercise

As a reward for your hard work these past two weeks, take a gentle stroll this evening and enjoy your alkaline body.

Treat

Get a reflexology massage. The massage focuses on reflex areas on your feet that are connected to parts of your body in order to relax these areas and open the energy flow. It promotes circulation and general healing.

'Modern life is acid. Accept it. See it for what it is and you can have your life back. You don't have to give up everything. You will just find some better alternatives, that is all. Enjoy it.'

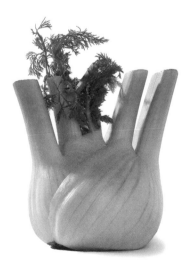

AFTER THE CURE

There are many things to take away after finishing the alkaline cure. Perhaps, after cleansing, you have lost some weight or you find yourself more agile physically and mentally. You may feel more supple, have fewer aches and pains. As you can see, a few small changes can have a dramatic effect and are more achievable than trying to change everything in an afternoon or even a month. Remember, a good regime is not just for fourteen days. The alkaline cure is a way of life, not a one-off detox. Keep going and you may surprise yourself with how good you can feel.

Hopefully you will have picked up enough tips to keep your system in balance, and hopefully you enjoyed it. Don't forget to slow down, chew well and really relish what you are eating. Listen to your body and eat only what will make your body feel good and healthy. Try to take exercise at least every other day – it doesn't matter so much what you do for exercise but rather that you exercise in the first place. And, in the whirlwind of everyday life, try to give yourself a good, manageable routine. With positive routines, your body will generate more power and energy.

A Regular Cure

Regularly repeating the alkaline cure will help you to establish a new self-understanding and build up your discipline. However, because you and your body have changed, your experiences each time around will feel slightly different.

The alkaline cure should become a part of your annual routine. It should be like – as it is for many people who come to the clinic each year – a summer holiday. 'Book' yourself back into the alkaline cure every year, but extend it to provide three weeks of cleansing. Hopefully by then many of the principles in this book will be an integral part of your everyday life, and you will be feeling the life-changing benefits.

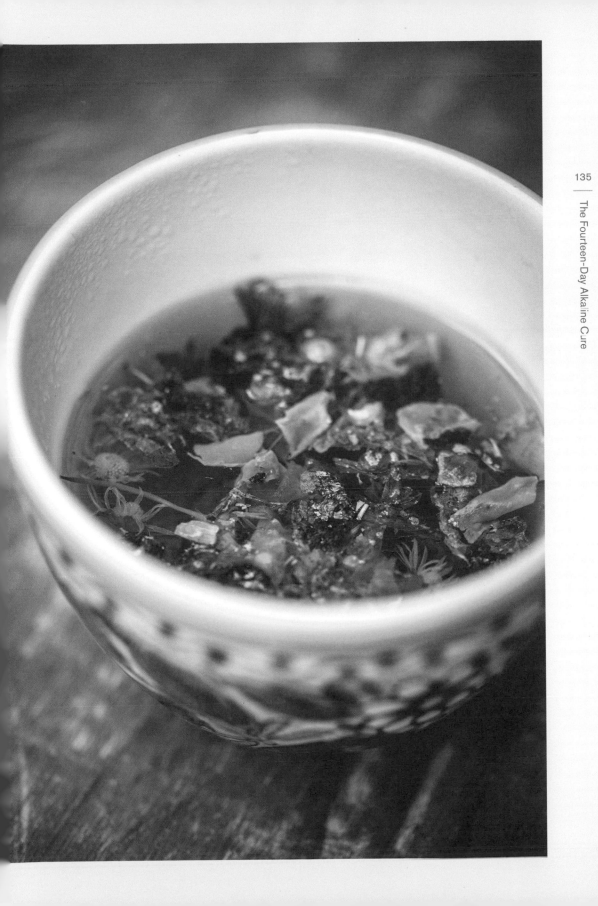

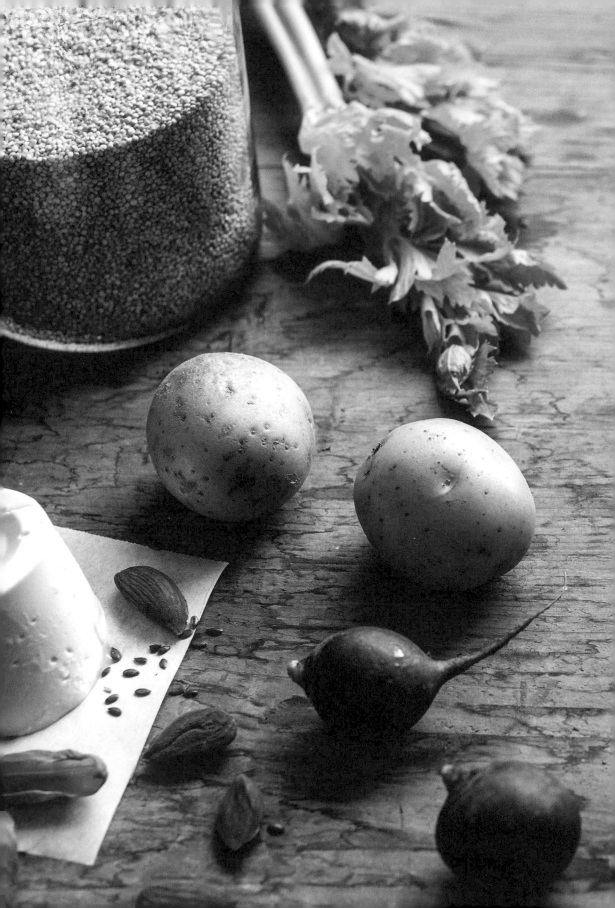

6

The Recipes

Teas and Infusions
Soups
Spreads
Breakfast
Lunch
Dinner
Oils, Sauces and Dressings

TEAS AND INFUSIONS

Teas and infusions are an excellent way of ensuring your body gets enough liquid throughout the day. They also offer many other health benefits. Though we recommend the teas listed here, there are many other great alkaline teas that you can substitute, such as rosehip, lavender, redbush and yerba mate. When making your own herbal tea infusions with fresh herbs or roots, simply add 235 millilitres of boiling water to one tablespoon of fresh herbs (or one teaspoon of dried herbs or grated root). Infuse the herbs for up to three minutes and strain.

MAYR VEGETABLE TEA

You can include the alkaline vegetables and spices according to the season. Rhubarb is a good addition, too, if you cannot find lovage. Drink this tea throughout the day to stay hydrated.

950 ml water
1 carrot, chopped
1 celery stalk, chopped
1 potato, chopped
Half a fennel bulb, chopped
1 broccoli stalk, chopped
Parsley stalks
1 teaspoon juniper berries

1 tablespoon chopped lovage
1 tablespoon chopped parsley
1 tablespoon fennel seeds
1 teaspoon coriander seeds
1 teaspoon cumin seeds
4 bay leaves

Put a large saucepan of cold water on to boil. Simmer the vegetables for ten minutes and then add the spices. Cover and simmer for 30 minutes. Turn off the heat. Leave to cool and infuse for another ten minutes.

Strain and keep the tea for use through the day – drink hot or cold.

MORNING TEAS

Your body is tuned to digest after a night's sleep. To get it started, a cup of hot water with (or without) a squeeze of lemon or lime first thing is the equivalent of rubbing the sleep out of your eyes. Drink this half an hour before breakfast. You can also enjoy the following morning teas to get you up and ready for the coming day.

Rosemary

Rosemary is an energising herb, known to promote blood circulation. It also stimulates digestion and improves cognitive function.

Ginger

Ginger tea is known for its ability to ease digestion and reduce nausea, but it has a number of other benefits as well. Packed with antioxidants, ginger also reduces inflammation, fights respiratory problems and relieves stress. Ginger increases blood circulation as well, which accounts for the warming sensation you experience when you drink it.

Thyme

Thyme is a remarkable herb. Not only can it clear chest congestion, relieve gas and bloating, and act as a diuretic, it is also full of antioxidants, vitamin K, and essential minerals, such as iron, manganese and calcium.

Sage

Sage is loaded with antioxidants. Antioxidants defend your body against harmful free radicals, which attack your cells and can lead to heart disease, cancer and premature ageing. Sage also relieves inflammation and treats gastrointestinal problems.

Peppermint

Peppermint tea is known to ease digestion and settle upset stomachs and nausea. It also contains calcium, vitamin B and potassium, which boost your immune system. Peppermint tea also has a calming effect and therefore is a great evening tea as well.

Nettle

Nettle has antiseptic and antimicrobial properties. It also contains many essential vitamins and minerals, such as iron, potassium and magnesium, as well as phytochemicals, which attack many of the free radicals that come from the environment. However, be careful not to consume too much nettle tea, as it can have an effect on blood sugar, blood pressure, anxiety, insomnia and blood clotting – especially if you are taking medication for any of these conditions.

Lemon Verbena

Lemon verbena has a calming effect on the nervous system and can even battle stress and symptoms of depression. The herb also aids digestion and helps relieve intestinal problems, such as nausea and diarrhoea.

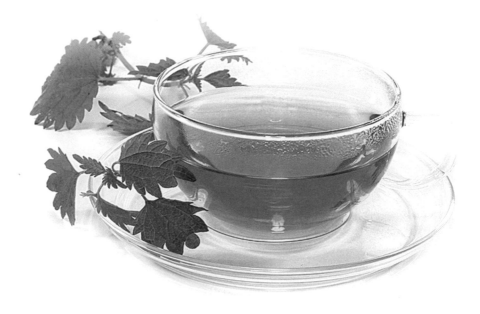

EVENING TEAS

After you've finished dinner and your daily tasks, relax and unwind with an evening tea. The following teas are known for their ability to ease digestion and calm your body, priming you for a good night's rest.

Lemon Balm
Lemon balm is a great evening tea because of its ability to calm. It treats everything from nervous agitation and digestive upsets to heart palpitations and viral infections. Lemon balm is also sleep-inducing, so try a cup before you turn in for the night.

Yarrow
Historically, yarrow was used for treating and healing wounds, but it has a number of other functions. Yarrow helps the body to sweat by relaxing the skin's pores and increasing blood circulation. It is also used to treat digestive problems; it stimulates the bowels and relieves gas and cramps.

Chamomile
Chamomile is best known as a sleep aid and, therefore, works well as a relaxing evening tea. It also soothes stomach and digestive upsets while regulating digestion. Chamomile is antibacterial and can be used to treat wounds and fight colds.

Fennel
You can make this tea with either the fennel's seeds, feathery leaves, roots or a combination of all three. It needs to be drunk right away to capture all the more volatile compounds before they evaporate. Fennel tea has long been known to ease digestive discomfort, relieving cramps and flatulence. It also acts as a diuretic, relieves pains and has antimicrobial properties.

SOUPS

Soup does not have to be just soup and you can make it more interesting by adding fresh herbs or flaxseed, nut or olive oils before serving. Liquidise soup to make it creamier and easier to digest. Soups are also useful for bringing important vegetables into your diet in different ways. They can be made the night before and either taken to work or reheated when you get home. And since soups need a bit of time to improve, it is a good idea to make them in advance.

Ⓥ ALKALINE MINESTRONE

This is our basic soup recipe, and the quantity is sufficient for a few days. It can be slipped into the diet for lunch or dinner. It is hearty, nutritious, healthy and delicious. By all means, vary the vegetables with the season and top up the soup with water you have used to cook other vegetables. This soup will last two or three days, and, if you eat nothing else, it is a big step forward to an alkaline way of life.

950 ml water or organic
   vegetable stock
1 medium potato,
   peeled and chopped
1 carrot, chopped
1 parsnip, chopped

1 turnip, chopped
1 celery stalk, chopped
50 g diced green onions
160 ml fresh cream
Rock or sea salt

Bring 950 millilitres of water or stock to a boil in a large saucepan, Add the chopped potato, followed by the other vegetables to the pot. Simmer for about 15 minutes, or until the vegetables are soft.

If you wish to liquidise your soup right away, turn off the heat and pour carefully into a food processor or use an electric handheld blender. Add the cream and the rock or sea salt to taste. Blend into a purée and garnish.

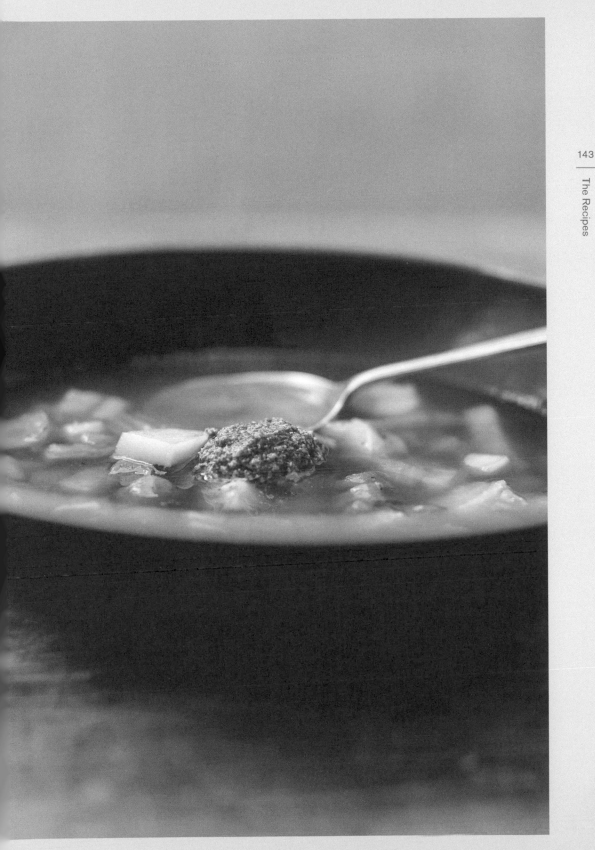

Ⓥ CELERY SOUP

1 head of celery, chopped	1 bunch parsley,
1 potato, peeled and	roughly chopped
chopped	Rock or sea salt
950 ml water	1 tablespoon curd

Chop the celery and potato into small chunks. Add the celery and potato to 950 millilitres of water and simmer for 20 minutes. Add the parsley stalks, keeping the leaves for a garnish.

When the vegetables are soft, remove from the heat and liquidise the soup in a food processor or using a hand blender until smooth. Season to taste with rock or sea salt. Scatter the parsley leaves over the soup along with a tablespoon of fresh curd.

Ⓥ HERB SOUP

Herb soups are a great way to maximise the benefits of the herbs you have in your garden or fridge, especially parsley, lovage and sorrel. The soup can also be filled out with a little spinach. In order to get a good, green colour, add the leaves in the food processor, without cooking. However, the stalks of parsley and coriander should go in at the start to flavour the broth. Use a good mix of herbs for this soup.

2 medium potatoes,	Herbs: parsley, basil,
peeled and chopped	chervil, lovage, coriander,
950 ml water or organic	thyme, rosemary
vegetable stock	Ground nutmeg
	Rock or sea salt

Boil the potatoes in water or vegetable stock until tender. Blend in a food processor or with an electric handheld blender. Add fresh herbs and blend again until the soup has a bright green colour. Add nutmeg and season with rock or sea salt.

ⓥ SPINACH AND NUTMEG SOUP

This is the fastest soup we know and it is also bursting with iron. You can give it new dimensions by adding herbs such as parsley, coriander or dill. You can probably also allow yourself a knob of butter or a touch of cream without upsetting the soup's alkalinity.

950 ml water or organic vegetable stock
450 g fresh organic spinach, washed
Rock or sea salt
Nutmeg

Bring the water or vegetable stock to a boil in a large saucepan. Add the spinach. Boil for one minute at most. Blend the soup in a food processor until smooth. Season to taste with rock or sea salt and a grating of nutmeg.

ⓥ LEEK AND POTATO SOUP

Leek and potato soup, sometimes called vichyssoise *when more cream is used, is both classic and also excellently alkaline. Traditionally, it is served cold in the summer and hot in the winter.*

2 tablespoons butter
1 medium onion, peeled
   and diced
4 potatoes, peeled and diced
4 leeks, finely chopped
950 ml water or organic
   vegetable stock

240 ml milk
Rock or sea salt
Pepper
Fresh chives or
   parsley, chopped
Cream or crème fraîche
(optional)

Melt the butter in a large saucepan and cook the onion until translucent, then add the potato and the leeks and stir well. After five minutes, add the vegetable stock and the milk, and cook for a further 20 minutes. Season with salt and pepper. Liquidise if you wish. Garnish with chopped chives, parsley or a spoonful of cream.

ⓥ CARROT AND GINGER SOUP

450 g carrots, washed
    and chopped
1 small potato, washed
    and chopped

700 ml water or organic
    vegetable stock
Ginger root
Rock or sea salt
1 orange
Parsley

Juice one-third of the carrots. Boil the remaining carrots and potatoes in vegetable stock or water until tender. Blend in a food processor until smooth. Grate in ginger to taste. Add the carrot juice and season with rock or sea salt. Add a squeeze of orange and garnish with parsley.

ⓥ FENNEL AND DILL SOUP

This soup is the original the recipe that Dr Mayr used to train patients to chew properly, served along with his famous spelt bread. It is simple and easy to make and very distinctive. This soup is to be eaten slowly. And be sure to be generous with the herbs.

950 ml water or organic vegetable stock
1 fennel bulb, quartered
1 bunch dill
Rock or sea salt

Bring the water or vegetable stock to a boil in a medium-sized pot. Dice three of the fennel segments and add to the water or stock. Juice the remaining segment and set aside.

When the fennel is cooked – just soft, about 12 minutes – add it to the food processor. Add in the fennel juice and the dill. Blend until smooth and season with rock or sea salt.

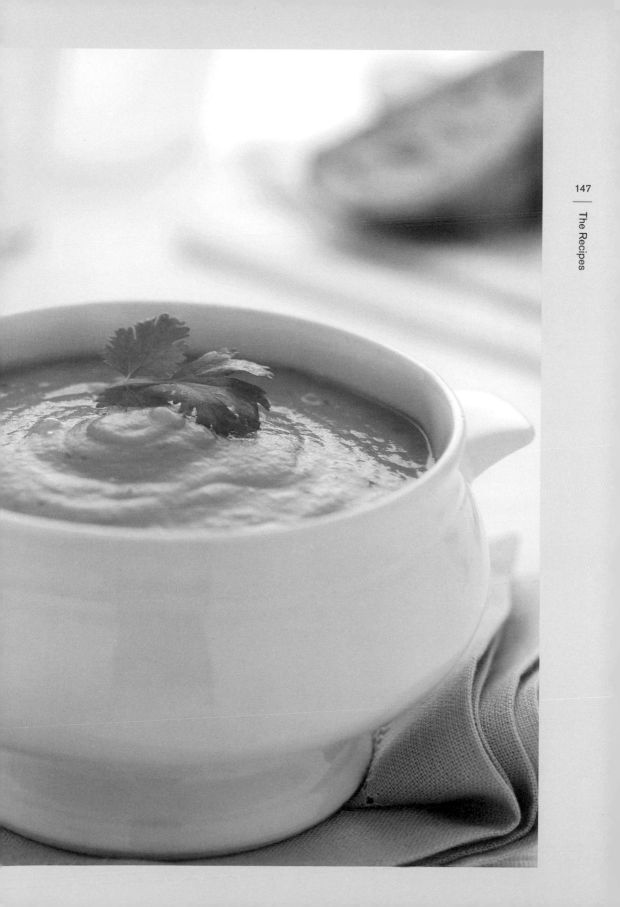

SPREADS

The following alkaline spreads are nutrient-dense alternatives to traditional breakfast spreads, such as jam or peanut butter, which can be both high in sugar and salt and loaded with preservatives. These spreads are versatile and easy to make, and the ingredients can be combined in countless ways. Enjoy the spreads over crispbread or spelt toast. Have one slice of crispbread or toast per meal and save the rest of the spread for the next day. You can substitute in quark, cottage cheese or probiotic yogurt if you don't have curd.

Ⓥ MEDITERRANEAN VEGETABLE SPREAD

One-quarter of a small
   aubergine, chopped
Half a courgette, chopped
45 g pitted black olives
60 g yogurt

150 g fresh, soft sheep's
   or goat's cheese
Rock or sea salt
2 tablespoons chopped basil
Olive oil

Heat a few drops of olive oil in a nonstick frying pan. Sweat the aubergine for two or three minutes. Then add the courgette and cook for a further two minutes. Blend in a food processor with the olives, yogurt and cheese. Season with rock or sea salt. Add the basil and a little virgin olive oil if needed.

Ⓥ SHEEP'S CHEESE AND HORSERADISH SPREAD

115 g fresh soft
   sheep's or goat's cheese
1 small potato,
   cooked and mashed

1 teaspoon grated fresh
   horseradish
1 teaspoon finely chopped
   fresh dill
Pinch of rock or sea salt

Blend all the ingredients in a food processor until very fine and season with rock or sea salt.

ⓥ CURD AND PAPRIKA SPREAD

55 g fresh curd cheese
1 tablespoon paprika
1 tablespoon flaxseed oil

Sprinkle paprika and drizzle flaxseed oil over the curd. Mix
to combine.

ⓥ HERB SPREAD

55 g curd or fresh, soft goat's
or sheep's cheese
1 tablespoon flaxseed or
olive oil
1 tablespoon finely chopped
parsley

1 tablespoon finely chopped
chives
1 tablespoon finely chopped
coriander
Paprika

Using the back of a fork, mash the curd or cheese with the flaxseed
or olive oil. Mix the herbs into the mashed curd. Dust with paprika.
Leave to stand for five minutes.

ⓥ AVOCADO SPREAD

2 ripe avocados
225 g fresh, soft sheep's
cheese
Juice of half a lime

1 teaspoon shredded basil
1 tablespoon sesame seeds
Pinch of rock or sea salt
Olive or pumpkin oil

Peel the avocados by cutting through the skin at quarter intervals and
peeling back the skin. Mash or blend the avocado flesh. Mix well with
the curd and the lime juice. Add the shredded basil and sesame seeds.
Season with rock or sea salt. Add a drizzle of virgin olive or pumpkin
oil. Serve immediately.

BREAKFAST

Breakfast can be one of the most important changes a person makes to their diet while on the alkaline cure. Breakfast should be a point where you bring in a wide range of different alkaline foods, particularly raw foods, because you have a whole day ahead to digest them. Spreads are a great way of doing this and, therefore, should become a regular breakfast staple as well. The following recipes typically serve one.

Ⓥ DRIED FRUIT POACHED IN HERBAL TEA

The alkaline triumvirate of dried apricots, figs and prunes can be given an extra boost by soaking them in herbal tea. They are a refreshing, nutritious hit to start the morning. You can drink the tea, too, which is delicious. Vary both the type of herbal tea and dried fruit, as you like.

190 g dried apricots, prunes or figs
1 tablespoon herbal tea of your choice
Water

Boil the water. Place the apricots, prunes or figs in a bowl. Pour over the boiled water. Add the herbal tea. Leave to cool and then store in the refrigerator overnight.

Ⓥ FRESH YOGURT WITH FLAXSEEDS

120 ml of fresh yogurt
1 tablespoon flaxseeds
1 tablespoon flaxseed oil

Sprinkle flaxseeds and drizzle flaxseed oil over the yogurt. Mix to combine.

Fresh Yogurt with Honey and Omega Mix
Sprinkle a tablespoon of omega mix (opposite) over the fresh yogurt. Sweeten with a teaspoon of honey. Make this breakfast more alkaline with the juice of a lemon.

ⓥ POWER MUESLI

Muesli can be difficult to digest so it is a good idea to soak it the night before in milk, apple juice, a thin yogurt, soy milk or almond milk. In the morning, mix with fresh fruit, soaked dried fruits (such as raisins), seeds, and nuts – especially almonds, for an even broader range of vitamins. This recipe will be enough for two or three breakfasts.

2 tablespoons oats
2 tablespoons millet flakes
2 tablespoons buckwheat
   flakes
235 ml almond milk, milk
   or apple juice
1 tablespoon currants
One-quarter of an apple

Half a carrot
2.5 cm piece of celery, diced
1 tablespoon sheep's
   yogurt
½ tablespoon walnut oil
½ tablespoon flaxseed oil
1 tablespoon crushed
   almonds

Soak the oats, millet and buckwheat in milk or apple juice. Add in the currants and leave overnight. In the morning, grate in the apple and carrot and add the diced celery. Top with the yogurt, oils and almonds.

ⓥ OMEGA MIX

You can get the benefits of seeds by creating your own mix in a coffee grinder or food processor. This mix is perfect for sprinkling on porridge, muesli, or salads.

3 parts flaxseeds
1 part pumpkin seeds
1 part sesame seeds
1 part sunflower seeds

Mix together and grind before use. You can store the mix in a jar and keep in either your store cupboard or fridge.

ⓥ MILLET AND BUCKWHEAT PORRIDGE WITH CINNAMON AND GINGER

This recipe is a simple variation on porridge that brings in some valuable spices.

25 g millet flakes	1 teaspoon ground
25 g buckwheat flakes	cinnamon
475 ml milk, soy milk	1 tablespoon grated ginger
or almond milk	1 tablespoon maple syrup

Soak the millet and buckwheat flakes in milk for at least ten minutes, but ideally overnight. Transfer to a pan and bring the porridge to simmering point, stirring and allowing it to thicken. Sprinkle with cinnamon and grate the ginger on top. Stir in the maple syrup.

ⓥ HERB OMELETTE

Eggs can be an easy source of protein, once or twice a week. The yolk is alkaline. Here, they are the perfect medium for fresh herbs.

Knob of butter	Half a bunch of parsley,
2 eggs	finely chopped
Rock or sea salt	Half a bunch of chives,
	finely chopped

Melt the butter in a nonstick frying pan. Break the eggs into a cup and beat with a pinch of rock or sea salt. Pour the beaten eggs into the hot frying pan. Once the omelette begins to set, sprinkle over the herbs, covering the omelette well. Fold over the omelette and leave to cook for a minute until set.

LUNCH

Lunch is the best time to explore a fuller range of alkaline ingredients. Your body still has sufficient time to digest properly and, therefore you are safe to incorporate both raw and cooked foods. The following recipes are much more interesting than a typical lunch, and far more alkaline, too. Each recipe typically serves one.

GRILLED CHICKEN WITH NEW POTATOES, BROCCOLI AND CARROTS

4 new potatoes, chopped
2 broccoli florets with
   their stalks
1 carrot, chopped
85 g chicken breast
2 tablespoons almonds

1 tablespoon butter
2 tablespoons chopped
   coriander
2 tablespoons chopped mint
Rock or sea salt

Turn on the grill to warm up. Trim the broccoli into florets. In a tiered steamer, put the potatoes on to steam first, then add the carrots and broccoli stalks. Grill the chicken for five minutes. Turn over and grill for a further five minutes. In a dry frying pan, toast the almonds quickly until they just begin to change colour – you can smell this happening.

After ten minutes add the broccoli florets to the potatoes and other vegetables. After a further five minutes, drain the vegetables, reserving the cooking water for minestrone stock or vegetable tea. Plate the grilled chicken.

Toss the vegetables in the butter and arrange them around the meat. Sprinkle the almonds over the broccoli, the coriander over the carrots and the mint over the potatoes. Season with salt.

ⓥ SALAD OF GREEN BEANS, POTATOES AND MIXED LEAVES IN OLIVE OIL

This is an easy, quick and nutritious lunch that is bulked up by the vegetables from your alkaline minestrone. You can vary the other vegetables as you like. Remember to top soups up with the cooking water from the vegetables.

1 small potato, washed and chopped

100 g green beans, trimmed

1½ tablespoons sunflower or sesame seeds

150 g mixed salad leaves

Pumpkin oil dressing (page 168)

75 g mixed vegetables from an alkaline minestrone (page 142)

Rock or sea salt

Place the potatoes in a tiered steamer. Steam for ten minutes. Add the beans to the potatoes, and steam for a further five minutes. Once cooked, set the potatoes and beans aside to cool. Toast the sunflower or sesame seeds quickly in a dry frying pan until they just begin to brown.

In a large bowl, toss the salad leaves with the pumpkin oil dressing. Mix the vegetables from your minestrone with the leaves. Top with the potatoes, green beans and roasted seeds. Sprinkle with rock or sea salt.

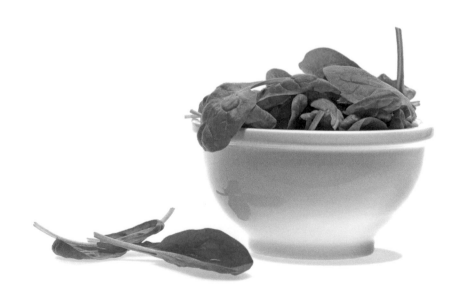

SEARED TUNA, AVOCADO, GINGER, CORIANDER AND LIME

Ginger root, peeled and grated
2 tablespoons chopped coriander
Half a lime
Rock or sea salt
Pepper
1 avocado, peeled, pitted and diced
Olive oil
85 g fresh tuna

Cover the bottom of a small mixing bowl with grated ginger. Add the coriander and lime juice. Mix well and season with salt and pepper. Add the avocado to the mix with a dash of olive oil.

Heat a frying pan on a high setting and sear the tuna for two minutes on either side, depending on its thickness. You can tell it is done when the colour of the fish has changed from dark to light. Serve the tuna on a plate with the avocado salad scattered over it.

FILLET OF BEEF WITH BRAISED CELERY AND MASHED SWEET POTATO

1 celery stalk, trimmed
Knob of butter
1 medium sweet potato, peeled and chopped
85 g fillet of beef
Black pepper
Horseradish

Place the trimmed celery in a pan and just cover with boiling water. Add the butter and braise slowly for 15 minutes.

In a second pan of boiling water, add the sweet potato and simmer for 15 minutes.

Preheat the grill. Once hot, grill the steak. Mash the sweet potato with a little butter and plenty of black pepper. Serve with horseradish.

ⓥ QUINOA SALAD WITH AVOCADO, TOMATO, PARSLEY AND PINE NUTS

You can use millet or bulgur wheat instead of all or part of the quinoa.

45 g quinoa
120 ml water
Handful of parsley,
  finely chopped

1 avocado, peeled, pitted
  and diced
Half a small tomato,
  chopped
Juice of half a grapefruit
10 pine nut kernels

Rinse and drain the quinoa. Add the quinoa and water to a saucepan and, over a high heat, bring the water to a boil. Once boiling, cover with a lid and reduce the heat to low. Cook for fifteen minutes, then remove from the heat. Fluff with a fork and allow to cool. Sprinkle the parsley, avocado and tomato over the top of the cooled quinoa. Pour the grapefruit juice over the quinoa and toss in the pine nut kernels.

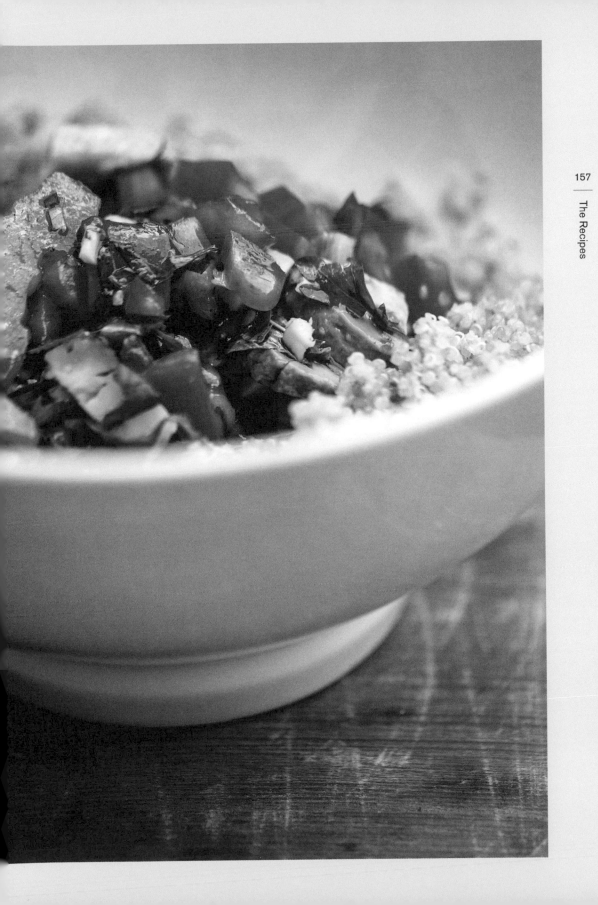

POACHED SALMON, CARROT AND SPINACH MASH, AND HEMP SAUCE

1 carrot
2 handfuls of spinach
Nutmeg
Ginger

Bunch of basil
Olive or hemp oil
Rock or sea salt
85 g salmon fillet

Poach the carrot for ten minutes until soft. Add the spinach for the last two minutes. Drain the carrots and spinach well, and mash them together with a little vegetable stock. Grate over the nutmeg and a little ginger.

In a blender, combine the basil leaves with a little olive or hemp oil and salt. The mixture should be vivid green and runny like a thin sauce.

Poach the salmon fillet in vegetable stock for two minutes. Serve the salmon on top of the mash and drizzle the green sauce on top.

Ⓥ ROASTED BEETROOT, BROAD BEANS AND CHIVES WITH WALNUT OIL

1 medium beetroot
55 g canned broad beans, rinsed and drained
3 tablespoons chopped chives
Walnut oil

Preheat the oven to 160°C. Wrap the beetroot in foil and bake for one hour. You can tell it is cooked when you can insert a knife easily. Set the beetroot aside to cool. When cooled, rub off the skin under cold running water. Shake dry and cut into several thick slices.

Add the broad beans to the beetroot and sprinkle the chives over the top. Dress with walnut oil.

ⓥ ASIAN-STYLE STIR-FRY

This is a recipe that we use at The Original F.X. Mayr Health Center because we have access to all these ingredients. You may want to simplify it a little to make at home. Commercial curry powders tend to be alkaline but if you don't like the spiciness you can substitute omega mix (page 151).

Coconut oil

5 cm piece of ginger root, peeled and crushed

1 stalk lemongrass, crushed and diced

2 shiitake mushrooms, chopped

1 small carrot, chopped

10 mangetout pods

One-quarter of a courgette, chopped

One-quarter of a leek, chopped

235 ml coconut milk

1 tablespoon curry powder

50 g soaked rice noodles or tofu (or both)

75 g long green beans, cut

1 pak choi

1 tablespoon coriander leaves

1 tablespoon Thai basil

Heat the coconut oil in a large wok. Add the ginger and lemongrass to the oil to flavour well. Add the vegetables to the wok, mixing well so they pick up the flavours. Add the coconut milk and the curry spice. Stir-fry for three minutes, then add the rice noodles or tofu. Cook for a further two minutes. Turn out into a bowl. Quickly boil the green beans and the pak choi together and add to the mix. Finish with the fresh herbs.

Ⓥ ARTICHOKE HEARTS WITH FLAXSEED AND HERB VINAIGRETTE

1 globe artichoke
Flaxseed oil or olive oil
Lemon

1 teaspoon mustard
1 tablespoon chopped
 fresh herbs

In a large pan, bring enough water to a boil to cover half the artichoke. Boil for 25 minutes or until the leaves come out easily.

Make up the vinaigrette with flaxseed or olive oil, a squeeze of lemon, a teaspoon of mustard and the herbs.

Eat the leaves first, one at a time. When you get to the base cut out the fine straw core and eat the artichoke heart with a little more herb vinaigrette.

This is a good recipe for teaching you to eat slowly.

Ⓥ BAKED PEPPER STUFFED WITH BULGUR WHEAT AND NUTS

75 g bulgur wheat
3 chestnuts, chopped
1 tablespoon pine nuts

1 tablespoon chopped
 parsley
Flaxseed oil or olive oil
1 red pepper

Preheat the oven to 160°C. To make the stuffing, pour boiling water over the bulgur wheat and simmer. Add the chestnuts and cook for 15 minutes. Strain the bulgur wheat and chestnuts, and mix in the pine nuts, parsley and a little oil to moisten.

Cut off the top of the pepper and remove the seeds. Fill the pepper with the stuffing. Bake the stuffed pepper for 20–25 minutes.

SPICY MEATBALLS WITH TZATZIKI

This recipe converts the usually (acidic) meatballs and tomato sauce into an alkaline treat by combining meatballs with a classic Greek yogurt sauce that is totally alkaline. All the other ingredients added to the minced beef – the onion, paprika, parsley and bread – are also alkalising, therefore lessening the acidity of the meat.

1 onion, diced

Coconut oil

85 g organic minced beef

1 egg

1 slice of bread, made into
   breadcrumbs

Paprika

Parsley, chopped

120 ml yogurt

75 g cucumber slices

3 garlic cloves, crushed

Mint, chopped

Fry the onion in coconut oil until translucent. Meanwhile, mix the meat with the egg, breadcrumbs, paprika and parsley (or other herbs). Add the onion to the meat mixture and roll into small balls. Put them into a frying pan to cook slowly.

To make the tzatziki, mix the yogurt with the cucumber slices, as much crushed garlic as you like and a generous handful of chopped mint. Serve with the meatballs.

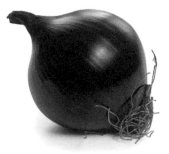

Ⓥ QUINOA RISOTTO

A quinoa risotto is easier to make than one made with white rice (and much more alkaline). Use the vegetables left over from an alkaline minestrone for this dish to add colour.

2 tablespoons curry powder
1 small carrot, diced
Half a celery stalk, diced
One-quarter of
   a courgette, diced
One-quarter of a sweet
   potato, diced

90 g quinoa, rinsed
1 tablespoon cashews
Lemon zest
3 tablespoons cream
   or soy cream
Basil leaves, torn

In a frying pan, dry roast the curry spices for a few minutes over a high heat until they start to release their oils. Add in the diced vegetables and mix well. Add 700 millilitres water and bring to a boil. Simmer for three minutes, then pour in the quinoa. Stir, keeping the mixture moving. Bring back to a boil and simmer for a further ten minutes.

While this cooks, toast the cashews in a dry pan until they start to colour. When the quinoa is cooked, add the lemon zest, cream (or soy cream) and cashew nuts. Garnish with fresh basil leaves.

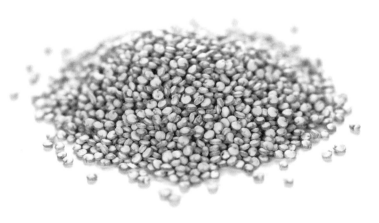

ⓥ GRATIN OF POTATOES, ONIONS AND NUTMEG

1 large potato, sliced

Half an onion, diced

Butter

Organic vegetable stock

Rock or sea salt

Pepper

Nutmeg

Preheat the oven to 180°C. Run the sliced potatoes under water to rinse off the starch. Lightly coat a baking tray with butter, and layer the potatoes and onions in it. Half cover with vegetable stock. Season with salt and pepper. Bake for one hour, until the top is crisp. Serve with a grating of nutmeg.

GRILLED LAMB CHOP WITH FENNEL, CUCUMBER, GRAPEFRUIT AND FIG SALAD

Add grapefruit to the salad if you have some left over from breakfast.

Half a fennel bulb, sliced

Half a cucumber, peeled and sliced lengthways

Half a grapefruit, segmented

2 fresh figs, cut open

2 tablespoons chopped mint

Parsley oil

1 lamb chop

Preheat the grill to high. Braise the sliced fennel in water for five minutes. Drain and place in a bowl with the cucumber slices, grapefruit, figs and mint. Put the lamb chop on to grill. Turn halfway through. The cooking time depends on how rare you like your meat.

DINNER

The earlier you have dinner, the better, as your body needs time
to digest fully before you go to bed. Portion sizes should also be
controlled for this same reason. A way to help you adjust your portion
sizes for dinner is by using smaller plates. We also recommend that
you avoid raw foods after four o'clock in the afternoon because they
are harder for your body to digest. A fully cooked vegetable soup is the
ideal way to round off your day, but the following recipes provide some
delicious, alkaline alternatives. Each recipe typically serves one.

Ⓥ BAKED POTATO WITH ALKALINE MAYONNAISE AND WATERCRESS

*A baked potato is such a dependable alkaline food that it deserves to be taken
seriously. You can also save the skins and fill with curd and herbs for a
quick lunch.*

>   1 baking potato
>   2 tablespoons alkaline mayonnaise (page 169)
>   1 tablespoon chopped watercress
>   Rock or sea salt

Bake the potato in the oven for about one hour, or until a knife slips in
easily. Take it out and set aside to cool slowly until you are ready to eat
– it will continue to cook in its own heat. To serve, slice the potato in
half and put one tablespoon of alkaline mayonnaise on each side and
garnish with the watercress and a sprinkle of rock or sea salt.

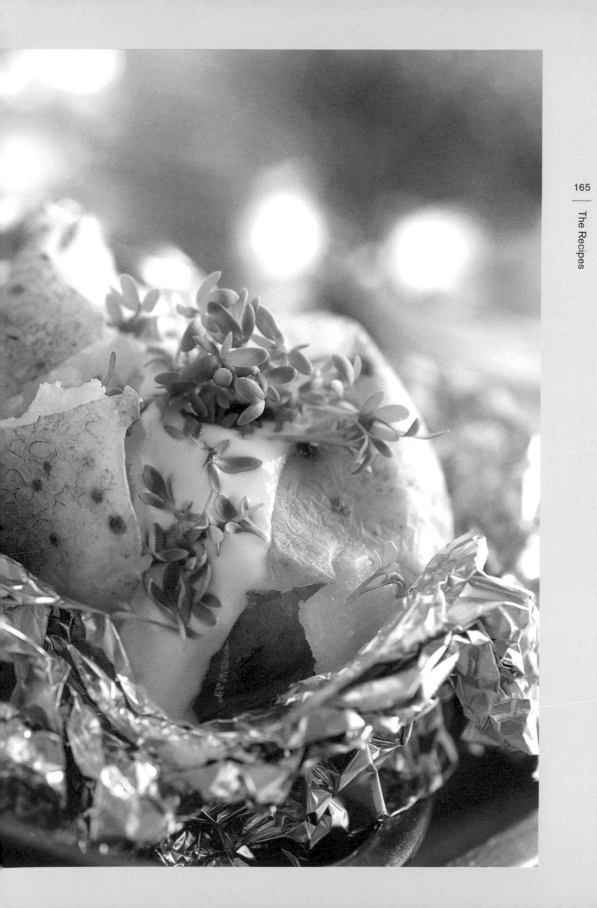

SMOKED MACKEREL AND VEGETABLES WITH PARSLEY OIL

This is a quick, easy supper if you are busy. You can substitute another smoked fish, such as smoked trout, if it is easier to find. Horseradish is alkaline but beware – many of the store-bought horseradish products are awash with acid ingredients.

85 g smoked mackerel fillet
Organic vegetable stock
200 g mixed vegetables
   from alkaline minestrone
   (page 142)

2 tablespoon parsley oil
1 tablespoon shaved
   horseradish

Warm through the mackerel in a little vegetable stock (or serve the fish cold).

Serve with the vegetables strained from an alkaline minestrone. Dress with parsley oil and shavings of fresh horseradish.

Ⓥ WARM SALAD OF KOHLRABI, BROCCOLI AND CELERIAC IN HERB OIL

This recipe is a bit of a shortcut because the cooking water from the vegetables can be used in a soup or as vegetable stock. Just add herbs and spices, and simmer for another ten minutes. You can vary the vegetables in this recipe but these go very well together.

Half a small kohlrabi, peeled and chopped
Half a small celeriac, peeled and chopped
1 large broccoli floret, cut into small pieces
2 tablespoons herb oil (page 168)

Simmer the kohlrabi and celeriac in a pan of water for ten minutes, then add the broccoli florets and cook for a further two minutes. Drain and reserve the cooking liquid. Serve the vegetables with herb oil.

ⓥ ROASTED BEETROOT WITH WALNUT OIL AND CARAWAY SEEDS

1 good-sized beetroot
Walnut oil
Caraway seeds

Preheat the oven to 160°C. Wrap the beetroot in foil and bake for 45 minutes to an hour, depending on size. When you can slip a knife easily through the middle, it is cooked. Leave to cool, then peel under cold running water.

Dress with walnut oil and sprinkle with caraway seeds.

ⓥ BRAISED FENNEL WITH COURGETTE

Half a fennel bulb, sliced
Half a courgette, sliced
1 tablespoon butter

1 tablespoon chopped
 parsley
Lemon

Slice the fennel lengthways. Place in the bottom of a small pan with just enough water to cover. Bring the water to a boil and cook slowly for ten minutes. Add the courgette and cook for a further five minutes. Make sure there is a little water left in the pan. Remove from the heat, add the butter, and garnish with parsley and a squeeze of lemon.

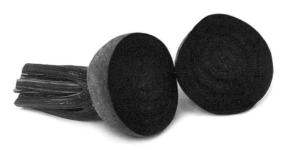

OILS, SAUCES AND DRESSINGS

Oils, sauces and dressings can help bring new flavour dimensions to seemingly plain dishes. Oils, particularly virgin oils, lend nutritional depth to your food as they are packed with vitamins and essential fatty acids. These oils, sauces and dressings are easy to make and much healthier than most store-bought sauces and dressings.

Ⓥ HERB OIL

Herb oils are an exciting way to get the value of the herbs into your diet in different ways. If you use parsley as a base you can add in other herbs for different textures, flavours and nutrients. Mix it up with flaxseed, pumpkin or nut oils for variety. This recipe makes 180 millilitres.

> Rock or sea salt
> 20 g flat-leaf parsley leaves
> 20 g tarragon leaves
> 175 ml extra-virgin olive oil

Bring a medium-sized saucepan of water to a boil. Add rock or sea salt to the water.

Blanch the parsley and tarragon (or other fresh herbs) until bright green – just ten seconds or so. Quickly drain and transfer to a bowl of iced water. Drain again and pat with a clean tea towel to remove as much water as possible. Blend in a food processor with the oil until smooth – at least a minute. Strain through a fine sieve or muslin.

You can keep the oil in the refrigerator for up to two weeks.

Ⓥ PUMPKIN OIL DRESSING

> 3 parts olive oil
> 1 part pumpkin oil
> 1 part lemon
>
> 2 tablespoons chopped
>   parsley or chives

Mix all of the ingredients together well and drizzle over a salad or vegetables.

ⓥ ALKALINE MAYONNAISE

Homemade mayonnaise can be a good vehicle for introducing flaxseed, pumpkin or nut oils into your diet. The yolk of the egg is alkaline (it is the whites that are acidic). This recipe makes about 700 millilitres.

1 egg yolk
1 teaspoon dry mustard
475 ml olive oil

120 ml flaxseed, pumpkin
  or nut oil
Rock or sea salt
Lemon

The egg should be at room temperature, and it is best if you use an old egg. Mix the yolk in a bowl with the mustard to form an emulsion. Slowly add the olive oil: stirring the mixture clockwise vigorously, add a small drizzle of olive oil until it is completely incorporated, then add a little more, and a little more. Finally, add the flaxseed, pumpkin or nut oil for flavour.

Season with salt and a squeeze of lemon.

ⓥ ALMOND PESTO

This dressing works well with the Alkaline Minestrone. This recipe makes about 80 millilitres.

1 basil plant
2 tablespoon almonds
2 tablespoons grated Parmesan
Olive, pumpkin, flaxseed or almond oil

Pick the leaves off of the basil plant. Put them in a blender with the almonds and Parmesan. Add two tablespoons of oil and blend.
If needed, add more oil to get a thick but manageable paste. Store in a jar and refrigerate; the pesto will keep for a week.

FREQUENTLY ASKED QUESTIONS

What if I work full time? Can I still follow the alkaline cure?
Absolutely. This is a very realistic goal. You can prepare your lunches
the day before and, if there are facilities available, warm them up at
work. However, it is important to try to cut down on stress during the
cure. It is therefore better to be at home during the programme and to
avoid travelling on business during that time.

If I don't eat meat, wouldn't that mean that I am naturally more alkaline?
Not necessarily. There are many vegetarian foods that are acidic as well
as generally unhealthy. For instance, vegetarian protein sources, such as
many types of cheese and soy, are acid-forming foods. Also, anything
alkaline that isn't chewed sufficiently will turn acidic in your stomach.
The key to an alkaline diet is to consider the balance and the quantity
of food you eat, and this applies to vegetarians and meat-eaters alike.

Can I have a glass of wine while I am on the cure?
During the fourteen-day plan it is best to give your system a complete
rest, so we advise no alcohol. Normally a glass of sherry or wine is no
problem – indeed it can even stimulate the digestive system – but it is
advisable to avoid sparkling wine, which is automatically more acidic.
Young wines tend to be less acidic than older wines.

Will I be hungry on the cure?
During the first week of the cure, you are likely to have one or two
days when you don't feel great. This is more likely the result of sugar
cravings than hunger. Try not to reach for the snack bar but do eat a
good breakfast, keep hydrated and get plenty of rest.

Why don't you have much fruit on the fourteen-day cure?
We like to minimise fibre consumption on the cure in order to be as
gentle on the stomach as possible. Fruit has a lot of sugar and can
ferment easily over the course of the fourteen days. Generally however,
fruit is fine in moderation so long as it is ripe. Often, the fruit we eat is
not ripe enough and this makes digestion harder.

What about eating out?
Restaurant menus generally tend to be acidic, although restaurants
that use fresh and good quality ingredients will likely offer some
alkaline dishes. Chain restaurants, for the most part, will have acidic
menus. If you go out and have a heavily acidic evening, just be aware of
the imbalance and remember to consume more alkaline foods in your
meals for the next few days. Soup is usually a good standby for this.

You recommend eating potatoes. Aren't potatoes fattening?
No – so long they are not deep-fried. They have more potassium than
bananas, have a high vitamins C and B6 content, and contain no fat.

I am on medication – is it safe to follow the alkaline cure?
Certainly – it will probably help. Many modern drugs upset the
bacteria in the stomach, so an alkaline diet may help you recover
quicker. However, you should check with your doctor before starting
this programme, if you are taking prescribed medication.

Can I be too alkaline?
Yes, but this is a rare condition and not connected to diet. If your pH
readings are very alkaline, see your doctor.

Can I be on an alkaline diet during pregnancy?
The general alkaline diet can be adopted and has been proven to
increase fertility. An alkaline environment is beneficial for an unborn
child, however we advise you to speak to a doctor before embarking on
the cure while pregnant.

Is the alkaline cure suitable for children?
This cure is not advised for children.

When is the best time to start the cure?
The best time is now.

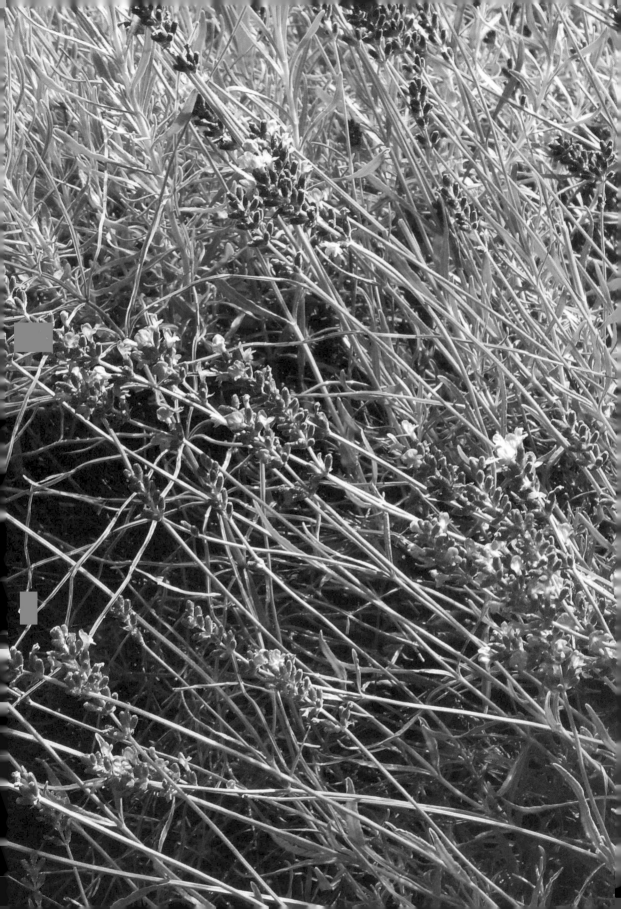

RECIPE FINDER

Teas and Infusions
Mayr Vegetable Tea 138
Morning and Evening Teas 139-141

Soups
Alkaline Minestrone 142
Celery Soup 144
Herb Soup 144
Spinach and Nutmeg Soup 145
Leek and Potato Soup 145
Carrot and Ginger Soup 146
Fennel and Dill Soup 146

Spreads
Mediterranean Vegetable Spread 148
Sheep's Cheese and Horseradish
    Spread 148
Curd and Paprika Spread 149
Herb Spread 149
Avocado Spread 149

Breakfast
Dried Fruit Poached in Herbal Tea 150
Fresh Yogurt with Flaxseeds 150
Power Muesli 151
Omega Mix 151
Millet and Buckwheat Porridge with
    Cinnamon and Ginger 152
Herb Omelette 152

Lunch
Grilled Chicken with New Potatoes,
    Broccoli and Carrots 153
Salad of Green Beans, Potatoes and
    Mixed Leaves in Olive Oil 154

Seared Tuna, Avocado, Ginger,
    Coriander and Lime 155
Fillet of Beef with Braised Celery and
    Mashed Sweet Potato 155
Quinoa Salad with Avocado, Tomato,
    Parsley and Pine Nuts 156
Poached Salmon, Carrot and Spinach
    Mash, and Hemp Sauce 158
Roasted Beetroot, Broad Beans and Chives
    with Walnut Oil 158
Asian-style Stir-fry 159
Artichoke Hearts with Flaxseed and
    Herb Vinaigrette 160
Baked Pepper Stuffed with Bulgur Wheat
    and Nuts 160
Spicy Meatballs with Tzatziki 161
Quinoa Risotto 162
Gratin of Potatoes, Onions and Nutmeg 163
Grilled Lamb Chop with Fennel, Cucumber,
    Grapefruit and Fig Salad 163

Dinner
Baked Potato with Alkaline Mayonnaise
    and Watercress 164
Smoked Mackerel and Vegetables with
    Parsley Oil 166
Warm Salad of Kohlrabi, Broccoli and
    Celeriac in Herb Oil 166
Roasted Beetroot with Walnut Oil and
    Caraway Seeds 167
Braised Fennel with Courgette   167

Oils, Sauces and Dressings
Herb Oil 168
Pumpkin Oil Dressing 168
Alkaline Mayonnaise 169
Almond Pesto 169

INDEX

acid food groups 67

acid-forming foods 19, 20, 68–69

acidity, excess 16–20, 36–37

acidosis 16, 36–37

ageing 16, 20, 29, 38, 41

alcohol 38, 69, 170

alkaline cure (fourteen-day
    plan) 94–135

alkaline food groups 70

alkaline-forming foods 19–20,
    71–78, 80–83

alkaline to acid rule 19, 30

allergies 24, 28, 76

antioxidants 72

balance, achieving 20, 21, 29, 30

bath soaks 107, 131

beansprouts 72, 78

beauty 21, 103, 107, 111, 115, 123,
    127, 131, 133

benefits of an alkaline cure 21–24, 39

bicarbonate of soda 54, 107, 115

bitterness 113

bloating 17

bones 17, 24, 29, 37, 66

bowels 22, 34

bread 28, 68, 86

breakfast 52, 150-152

breathing exercises 107, 121, 127

caffeine 69

candida 68, 77, 78

carbohydrates 21, 64

chewing 33, 47, 48–49, 104

cleansing the system 57, 100–115, 170

constipation 17, 22

cooking 90–93

dairy 66, 67, 68, 86

dental health 17

diabetes 28

digestive system 32–34, 36–37,
    38, 52, 53

dinner 52, 164-167

disease 17, 19, 25, 28, 41

dressings 168-169

dried fruit 75, 87

energy and vitality 17, 21, 22

environment 59, 105, 109, 113,
    121, 125, 129

enzymes 32

Epsom salts 57

exercise 56, 98, 133

cardio 56, 103, 111, 125, 131

strengthening 109, 123, 129

stretching 105, 113

face mask 127

fats 66, 67, 69, 88–89

fermentation 36–37

fertility 24

fish 28, 68, 86

foot bath 115

frequently asked questions 170–171

fruit 37, 50, 69, 70, 74–75, 83, 86

gargling 98

gluten 76

grains 64, 70, 75–76, 82, 86, 87

hair mask 103

herbs 70, 77, 86, 92, 139-141, 144

hydration 54–55, 64, 98

intestines 34

kitchen equipment 85

lifestyle 28–31, 41

liver compress 123

lunch 52, 151–161

Mayr, Dr Franz Xaver 12–13, 39,
    57, 68

MBSR (Mindfulness Based
    Stress Reduction) 46

meat 17, 66, 68, 84, 86

mental health 22, 46

mindful eating 46–47, 49

minerals 37, 50, 55, 66, 72, 77, 121

nuts 67, 70, 81, 87

obesity 17, 28, 29

oils 66, 70, 82, 87, 88–89

    cooking with 89

    and dressings 168-169

    gargling with 98

    refined 69

overeating 36–37, 53

pH testing 14–15

portion control 53

preserving foods 93

processed foods 21, 28, 29, 39, 67, 93

protein 20, 66, 67, 68

raw foods 37, 52

Recipe Finder 173

reflexology massage 133

rest and recuperation 60, 61

rhythm of life 60–61

root herbs 77–78, 81, 139

saliva 15, 33, 49

salt 92

salt scrub 111

seeds 78, 80, 87

shopping 86–87, 100–101, 118–119

skin 17, 21, 37, 38, 98

sleep 17, 21, 52, 125

soups 142 147

spices 78, 87, 92

spreads 148–149

stomach 33, 38, 57

store cupboard basics 87

stress 38, 46, 60

sugar 38, 64, 69

superfoods 80–83

teas and infusions 138-141

temperature, body 61

timing of meals 52, 60

vegetables 50, 70, 71–74, 86, 93

    cooking 90

    raw 37, 52

    superfoods 80, 81, 82, 83

vitamins 66, 71–72, 77

water 54–55, 64, 98

weight loss 22, 25, 30

Western diet 31

whole foods vs purées 93

ACKNOWLEDGEMENTS

I would like to say thank you to Drew for his unbelievable help, patience, good spirits and wisdom; to Silvia and the team at Elwin Street for the opportunity; to Ilana Stein for her support; to Margo Marrone at The Organic Pharmacy; to all my patients who have helped me learn; to my teachers Dr Schulz, Dr Stossier and Dr Werner; and, last but not least, to my wife and my children for all of their support and love.

Elwin Street would like to thank everyone at The Original F.X. Mayr Health Center for their help in creating this book, Drew Smith for his contributions and Alessandra Spairani for her beautiful photography.

Resources

To purchase base powder and other alkaline health products, please visit The Organic Pharmacy at www.theorganicpharmacy.com.

To purchase pH litmus strips, please visit Micro Essential Inc. USA at www.microessentiallab.com.

For more information about *The Alkaline Cure*, please visit www.thealkalinecure.com.

For more information about the companion recipe book *The Alkaline Canteen* and for more delicious alkaline recipes, please visit www.thealkalinecanteen.com.

For more information about The Original F.X. Mayr Health Center, please visit www.original-mayr.com.

Photo Credits

Alessandra Spairani: pp. 10-1, 23, 26-7, 35, 39, 42-3, 51, 62-3, 65, 73, 79, 91, 94-5, 99, 117, 135, 136-7, 143, 157; Dreamstime: pp. 89, 103, 140, 167; Drew Smith: pp. 18, 40, 58, 172; Getty: pp. 55, 74, 147, 165; iStock: pp. 7, 13, 30, 45, 49, 84, 101, 105, 107, 108, 111, 112, 115, 119, 120, 123, 125, 126, 128, 131, 133, 154, 161, 162; The Original F.X. Mayr Health Center: pp. 3, 8